SPECIAL NEEDS KIDS are people too!

SEEING THE POSSIBILITIES THROUGH A NEURODIVERSE LENS

by Amy Bodkin, EdS
Autistic Adult & Special Needs Consultant

Copyright © 2024 Amy Bodkin Consulting LLC. All rights reserved.

No part of this book may be reproduced in any form or by any electronic or mechanical means, including information storage and retrieval systems, without permission in writing from the publisher, except by reviewers, who may quote brief passages in a review. For permission requests, contact the author at: support@amybodkin.com.

Amy Bodkin is an Autistic adult, Consultant, and Public Speaker serving families with needs that fall outside the norm. Amy has an Educational Specialist degree in Educational Psychology with an emphasis in Neuropsychology, a Master's degree in Educational Psychology, and she homeschools her two Autistic children. Her business, Amy Bodkin Consulting, serves both families and professionals by providing educational resources, private consultations, workshops, and more.

Visit Amy Bodkin at AmyBodkin.com.

Library of Congress Cataloging-in-Publication Data
Bodkin, Amy, author.
Lebowitz, Rachel, editor.
Special needs kids are people too : seeing the possibilities through a neurodiverse lens / by Amy Bodkin, EdS.
Description: Includes bibliographical references and index. | Corpus Christi, TX: Neurodiverse Press, 2024.
Identifiers: LCCN: 2024908712 | ISBN: : 979-8-9905128-3-2 (hardcover | 979-8-9905128-0-1 (ebook) | 979-8-9905128-1-8 (audio)
Subjects: LCSH Neurodiversity. | Children with disabilities--United States. | Learning disabled children--Education. | Autistic people. | Autism in children. | Autistic children--Education. | Developmentally disabled children. | Children with autism spectrum disorders. | Parents of developmentally disabled children. | PSYCHOLOGY / Developmental / Child | EDUCATION / Inclusive Education | FAMILY & RELATIONSHIPS / Children with Special Needs
Classification: LCC HV1570.25 .B63 2024 | DDC 616.85/882--dc23

Contents

Introduction   v

Part One
Philosophical Underpinnings

1. Towards a Philosophy of Practice   3
2. Why Special Needs?   9
3. Towards a Philosophy of Education   17
4. Towards a Psychology of Being   27
5. The Power of Myth and Personal Transformation   37
6. The Power of a Story   47
7. The Humanities: A Roadmap to Inner Peace   55

Part Two
Practical Application

8. Development: A Roadmap to Education   65
9. Physiological Needs are More Than Just Skin Deep   75
10. Safety Needs = Self Care   83
11. Self-Esteem = Love and Belonging   93
12. Cognitive and Aesthetic Needs = Seeing the Beauty that is All Around Us   105
13. Self-Actualization and Transcendence   117
14. Putting It All Together: Case Studies   127

    About the Author   143
    Other Resources by Amy Bodkin   145
    Charlotte Mason's 20 Principles   147
    Works Cited   153
    Bibliography   155
    Index   159
    Disclaimer   161

Introduction
Special Needs Kids Are People Too

Thank you for purchasing this book! And welcome to a journey that I believe is worth taking: seeing the possibilities through a neurodiverse lens.

I'm Amy Bodkin, an Autistic School Psychologist, and I have homeschooled both of my Autistic children since the beginning. I have an Educational Specialist Degree (EdS) with an emphasis in Neuropsychology, a Master of Science degree in Educational Psychology, and a Bachelor of Science degree in Psychology with a minor in Mathematical Sciences.

Personally, professionally, and as a parent, I have a significant amount of experience with Autism and all the many processing and learning disabilities that can go with Autism, as well as many other types of diagnoses. All of these different angles of experience give me a very unique perspective and insight into not just education but also how we, as a society, treat students who fall outside the average.

To See a Child as a Person, not a Diagnosis

Too often, children with "special needs" are viewed as "less than" because of their differences. As a consultant, I make it my business to see each child as an individual and not as a diagnosis. And as an advocate, I encourage others to do the same.

Rethink the way life "has to be" and try instead to envision how it "could be." Too many times people only see "deficits" and what they "don't have to work with." I would like to encourage people to start thinking about the wonderful person each child already is and what supports will fit their needs best. Create an atmosphere that allows all people to be who they were born to be, so we can all stop trying to "fake it till you make it."

Seeing the Possibilities Through a Neurodiverse Lens

This book lays out the philosophy that I have developed to guide my practice both as a professional and as a parent. As such, this book has been designed for use by both professionals and parents. The first half guides you through discovering those who influenced the development of my philosophy of practice. The second half of the book guides you through the application of my philosophy of practice.

My goal is to help children find more balance. When a child ends up developing one skill in abundance to his other skills, we can end up with some rather unfortunate consequences. Van Gogh, Beethoven, etc., were all extremely talented in their fields, but if there is one thing you notice about some of the most talented people, it is that they are often not very happy. People need balance to gain confidence and contentment. And isn't that what we want for children? For them to grow into confident and contented adults?

Practical Application

There is no way I could possibly include everything in one book. So I contented myself with focusing on the philosophy behind what I do. However, if you would like practical help in a specific area, I am in the process of creating more educational resources, what I call "Boost Packets," on my website that dive into specific and practical topics related to this book. I also offer a membership as well as one-on-one consultations for those needing more personalized assistance.

More Ways to Connect

If you have questions about this book or would like to connect further, visit my website at AmyBodkin.com or scan the QR code below to get access to free book discussions offered periodically throughout the year. There is a book discussion for parents and another one for professionals so that everyone will benefit from a discussion that is tailored to their needs.

And please, share this book with others! What a wonderful world this would be if we all recognized that Special Needs Kids are People Too!

Amy Bodkin, EdS
Autistic Author, Speaker, and Consultant
AmyBodkin.com

Scan the QR code for more information about our live book discussions at AmyBodkin.com!

Part One

Philosophical Underpinnings

Chapter 1

Towards a Philosophy of Practice

"A recipe has no soul. You, as the cook, must bring soul to the recipe."
- Thomas Keller

After many years, my experiences as an Autistic child, my training as a School Psychologist, and my experiences homeschooling my two Autistic children eventually simmered together long enough that they melded into a unique flavor of my very own.

Over the last several years, I have been honored to share that special blend with parents and professionals through hundreds of individual consultations. Like the response of satisfied diners, their reactions have helped me realize what a gift I was sitting on, and as Tiana's father in *The Princess and the Frog* put it upon tasting his daughter's gumbo, "A gift this special just got to be shared!"

As an Autistic child who grew into an Autistic adult, I have experienced what it feels like to not fit in, to live in a society not designed for me. I know what it feels like to have an Auditory Processing Disorder (APD), to be Dyslexic, to experience sensory overload, to have meltdowns, and to have panic attacks.

I also know the joys of special interests, the satisfaction of stims, the importance of honesty, and having a friend who understands you!

I was not always able to express these things. Despite having the ability to "talk to a wall," it was not until well into adulthood that I had enough cognitive development to be able to reflect on my experiences introspectively and then to be able to give expression to those experiences. As suggested in the book *Jane Eyre* by Charlotte Bronte, "Children can feel, but they cannot analyze their feelings; and if the analysis is partially affected in thought, they know not how to express the result of the process in words."

One of the few executive functioning skills I did fully develop is meta-cognition, which means I am very good at seeing patterns. Having the ability to see patterns well and having all of these different lived experiences has given me much more insight into understanding myself and others like myself than is typically available in the research. Unfortunately, the vast majority of funded research is focused on how to fix or to cure Autistics with early intervention or treatments, which on the whole, isn't very helpful. We would much prefer research focused on improving our quality of life.

The average life expectancy for an Autistic is only 36 years old due to accidental death, suicide, autoimmune conditions, and sometimes murder.[1,2,3] The average life expectancy of a neurotypical adult is approximately 72 years of age, meaning an Autistic's average life expectancy is half that of the average adult. And there are quite a few research topics in the area of improving quality of life as well as potentially improving life expectancy available, but few have undertaken any of this research.

As a School Psychologist, I obviously received the appropriate training in research, behavior, assessment, academic intervention, child development, law, and ethics. However, I also received additional training in neuropsychology and statistics. When it comes to practical experience, I obtained a substantial amount through my work in public schools, private school consulting, and private practice.

Generally speaking, private schools were not nearly as well equipped to handle students with different needs or even know where problems might exist. But they were often willing to do what they could to accommodate a student if possible.

In public schools, there were always several outstanding teachers that genuinely cared, but I also saw a lot of corruption. I get Individualized Education Plans (IEPs) across my desk from all over the United States. What strikes me about these supposedly SMART (Specific, Measurable, Achievable, Relevant, and Time-bound) goals is that they continually inform us about what the student will do, not usually what the district promises to do for the student. By examining who the IEP goals truly safeguard, you can catch a glimpse of the corruption I witnessed.

However, corruption doesn't always originate from within the school administrative system. Sometimes it comes into the school from the students' homes and community.

One of the worst things I noticed was middle school male special education students being targeted for sexual assault by neurotypical middle school female students. Students as young as fifth grade told me that getting pregnant meant possibly receiving a welfare check, and that if they "beat the kid until they were stupid," they could also possibly get an additional stipend in the form of a "crazy check," so choosing a father in special education was advantageous. What was even worse was that the male assault victims were often the ones punished by the school system.

Witnessing things like this is one of the major reasons I chose to leave public education. It was simply too heartbreaking to watch these things happening day after day and feel so limited in what I could do about it.

Now, as a parent, I have even more compassion for children being failed by any system.

Having my own children has been a fascinating experience! Since both of my children are also Autistic, for the first time in my life, I have had the opportunity to live with other Autistics like me, and it has been such a source of joy in my life! But I also learned a lot because they differ significantly from me in their strengths and weaknesses. We also experienced interesting challenges in the area of communication development with my youngest. These challenges led me to learn about an entire category of differences in development and learning that I had not even heard about in graduate school. And none of the many speech therapists I took him to in our area had ever heard of a child who taught himself to read by the time he turned two years old, which we now know was Hyperlexia. These days, more professionals are likely to have come across the term Hyperlexia, but it remains relatively obscure and is likely not covered in graduate programs.

As a parent, I also developed a great deal of compassion for other parents. I could now understand the trauma of wanting to be the best parent for your child while also feeling overwhelmed by the long lists of professional recommendations that can feel impossible. The sense of inadequacy you sometimes feel as a parent can be overwhelming, not to mention exhausting.

When we decided to homeschool our children, once I had gotten over the initial panic of becoming solely responsible for my children's education, I eventually learned to trust my children more than my own expertise. They are the only ones in their bodies and the only true experts on themselves. If I only simply observe their verbal and nonverbal communication, they are already trying to tell me what they need. And like plants, they will learn and grow when they are ready to, so long as I provide them with a well-balanced diet, physically, mentally, and emotionally.

I have also learned as a homeschool parent (due to the large amounts of time we spend with our children) that while I may not be my children's best friend, I should treat them with the same respect I would give to my best friend. And if I can do that, we will have smooth and easy days even during turbulent times.

Throughout this book, you will see hints of how my varied experiences have congealed to create a philosophy of practice uniquely my own, and I will introduce you to three authors whose ideas have greatly influenced me and now represent my experiences as a Homeschool Parent, School Psychologist, and Autistic individual respectively. These three authors have not been my only influences, but they have been the most meaningful.

There are two parts of this book: Philosophical Underpinnings and Practical Application.

In Part 1, Philosophical Underpinnings, you will find references to all of my "special interests," from Science Fiction and Mythology to Patanjali's Yoga Sutras. Each one of my special interests is relevant as each has served as an ingredient in my educational recipe for supporting struggling children. You, of course, do not have to agree or even like my special interests to benefit from this book. But it is my hope that taking this journey with me will give you the necessary catalyst for change regarding how we view and relate to struggling children.

In Part 2, Practical Application, I will walk you through the process I use in each of my consultations to determine the order and method that will provide the most significant gains for children with the least amount of effort from their parents!

While my goal in writing this book is to help parents help themselves and encourage professionals to shift their approach and goals, this book will not be a standardized recipe full of steps and measurements. The best cooks know that something special is lost in the standardization of a recipe. It is not the consistent measurement of ingredients that makes food taste good. It is the relationship between the cook, the flavors, the process, the presentation, and even the people she shares it with. Or as Thomas Keller said, "A recipe has no soul. You, as the cook, must bring soul to the recipe."

With that in mind, I will take you on a journey through the relationships and interactions that came together to create my recipe. And even though applying this educational recipe to different children doesn't always look the same or have the same ingredients, it always honors a child's individuality and supports the child in his next developmental steps.

And "You know the thing about good food?" as Tiana's father so eloquently put it in *The Princess and the Frog*, "It brings folks together from all walks of life. It warms them right up, and it puts little smiles on their faces."

That is how I hope you will experience this book, and when you share my educational recipe with others, I hope that it will put "little smiles" on their faces and "warm them right up."

Chapter 2

Why Special Needs?

"Part of the problem with the word 'disabilities' is that it immediately suggests an inability to see or hear or walk or do other things that many of us take for granted. But what of people who can't feel? Or talk about their feelings? Or manage their feelings in constructive ways? What of people who aren't able to form close and strong relationships? And people who cannot find fulfillment in their lives, or those who have lost hope, who live in disappointment and bitterness and find in life no joy, no love? These, it seems to me, are the real disabilities."
- Fred Rogers

Since I started using the term "special needs" for my work, I have taken a lot of flak for it from fellow Autistics, professionals, and parents. People often ask questions like, "Why don't you use neurodivergent?" or "Why don't you use exceptional?" And I have honestly given this a lot of thought because if I am going to run counter to what everyone is telling me, then I need to have a good reason and know why I disagree with everyone else!

So, why not use neurodivergent? I use it all the time to

describe myself, so why not use it in my work? The reason is that I work with families who do not always fit neatly into the description of neurodivergence.

The definition for *neurodivergence*, according to *The Oxford Dictionary*, is "divergence in mental or neurological function from what is considered typical or normal."

But this definition doesn't always fit children with a physical disability or a severe medical condition, a parent with an autoimmune disease, adopted children, foster children, or one of the many other situations requiring special care. Of course, some of these situations may lead to a difference in neurology, but that doesn't mean those individuals are ready to self-identify as neurodivergent. Sometimes they have to mourn the loss of their own previously held expectations of who they were and how the future might look. Sometimes they just have to recognize and acknowledge their legitimate feelings before they are ready to take on a new moniker and, indeed, a new identity!

Then why not use exceptional? It sounds so positive! We get the opportunity to highlight how everyone has things that make them excellent!

The definition of *exceptional* according to *The Oxford Dictionary* is "unusually good or very unusual." But in educational settings, the term *exceptional* has been, more times than not, used to describe children who are identified as gifted. This brings up a completely different set of word problems.

In the United States, giftedness is an educational identification based on a student's Intelligence Quotient (IQ). Most people's experience with IQ scores is that they measure one's intelligence, which would make sense. Except, that is not correct.

In the late 19th century and early 20th century, psychologists explored the concept of intelligence and endeavored to develop a method for measuring people's intelligence. Eventually, they were able to develop a test that they thought could gauge intelligence, what we now know as a standard IQ test. The belief was so strong that the United States military used these tests on a mass scale during World War I to determine which enlistees should be selected as officers. Of course, that led to a large amount of data that could then be used for further research on intelligence. This also led to the unfortunate and inaccurate conclusion by researchers that certain ethnic groups were more intelligent than others.[1] This, of course, was not true but was a bias in the test.

This further led to the United States Supreme Court upholding the right of the government to force sterilization on citizens with low IQ scores (Buck v. Bell, 1927).[2] This, then, resulted in a more significant percentage of people of color being forcibly sterilized than their white counterparts. While eugenics has somewhat fallen out of favor, the Supreme Court's decision has never been overturned.

We have learned from intelligence testing over the last century that despite our most audacious dreams, IQ tests do not actually measure intelligence. Like the people of old endeavoring to build a tower to the heavens, we also thought ourselves equal to the Divine. And, like them, we, too, have been humbled. This doesn't mean that intelligence tests are entirely useless. They can offer valuable insights into how a person processes information at a particular moment; however, they cannot, and never have been able to, predict future ability.

As you can see, intelligence tests have been used to separate people into those who are "valuable" and those who are not. They have also been used to divide students between those deserving of an enriching curriculum and those pulled from all elective subjects for remedial assistance in reading and math. And the reality is that there is no basis for such decisions.

I once had a teacher in high school who told my class that one year she had been given her class roster, and each student had a number next to their name. As she looked at the numbers, she concluded that they must be her students' IQ scores and that she had better do an outstanding job teaching this year to live up to her students' potential. She later found out that those numbers were their locker numbers, but it taught her a valuable lesson about the power of our perceptions.

It's important to note that gifted students also face unique challenges due to their atypical development. But we have a tendency to minimize the challenges of gifted students and only focus on their strengths. Likewise we also have a tendency to minimize the gifts of students with learning disabilities and tend to focus solely on their challenges. It is ignorant to label giftedness positively and learning disabilities negatively. Both identifications represent imbalances in development, and each comes with its own set of strengths to celebrate and weaknesses to support.

A similar effort to categorize has been happening to Autistics as well as within the Autistic community. Until recently, children considered "higher functioning" were diagnosed with Asperger's Syndrome, while children considered "lower functioning" were diagnosed as Autistic. Even though the Asperger's diagnosis no longer exists, many people still choose to identify themselves as having Asperger's. Why is that? Some people prefer to stick with Asperger's because it was the diagnosis they were given. But, sometimes, people stick with Asperger's to separate themselves from "lower functioning" Autistics. And there can be reasons to do this as it can affect how others, especially those in authority, may judge you.

However, some opt to identify as Autistic to unite their voices and advocate for the greater good of the Autistic community. Others choose to identify as Autistic due to the complicated legacy of Hans Asperger, the man for whom Asperger's is named.

The first time anyone discussed Autism was in the late 1930s when Hans Asperger spoke to Nazi officials about the unique abilities of some of his Autistic patients, though they were not yet called Autistic. Was he acting as a willing agent of the Nazis by doing their dirty work deciding which children had value to the state and which did not and should be sent to the first death camps? Or was he working as an undercover operative doing what he could to preserve lives? The world may never know for sure, as the motivations of a man's heart go with him to the grave. What we do know is that the complicated history of Autism, including Hans Asperger himself, continues to have an impact on the words we choose today. You can learn more about this fascinating history in the book *Neurotribes: The Legacy of Autism and the Future of Neurodiversity* by Steve Silberman.

The words we use matter. So why not use the term exceptional? As you can see from the examples of intelligence testing and Asperger's, exceptionalities have been used to separate people into those who have real value and those who don't. That does not inspire a sense of equality or brotherhood. However, recognizing that we all have struggles, weaknesses, and needs unites us as we realize what we have in common as human beings. We all struggle in some way, at some point, because that is how growth happens, and that is what it means to be a living being, to constantly be in a state of growth and change. In fact, only when we stop growing and changing do we go from living to dying.

The challenges we all experience vary significantly from person to person, and it almost always diverges from the nonexistent "golden average." So why not change the term from "special needs" to "human needs?"

The Oxford Dictionary defines *special* as "not ordinary or usual; different from what is normal."

In truth, many of these needs are special in that they are outside the norm and not naturally accommodated for, while other needs are more common and thus naturally accommodated for.

In an ideal world, all needs would be taken into account as "human needs" without this emphasis on a diagnosis proving their necessity. In fact, many accommodations work equally well, if not better, for people without a diagnosis. However, in our less-than-perfect world, I suspect that, in some ways, a drive toward "human needs" would eventually denigrate the real struggles of very real, though not typical, needs that are not being accommodated.

Trying to emphasize that these are all just "human needs" could also allow us to identify our needs in a way that says, "I'm not different. I'm just like everybody else." And why would it be a problem to see no difference? We are, after all, members of the same human race. But it is a problem. We have learned over recent decades that being color-blind to racial differences does not lead to true inclusivity. In fact, it does quite the opposite and bars us from celebrating what is truly beautiful and valuable about our differences, shaped by our unique journeys.

There is an episode of *Star Trek: The Next Generation* (yes, I'm a Trekkie!) in which the Genome colony risks annihilation because their carefully engineered society cannot easily be separated from their planet. It turns out that the solution was found in a piece of technology worn by Geordi, the Chief Engineer of the Starship Enterprise, a blind man. The VISOR (Visual Instrument and Sensory Organ Replacement) he wore provided him with a sense of sight. But he never would have been born in the Genome colony because his existence was not valued. And yet, it was his very existence and the technology created to support his need that protected the Genome colony from extinction.

We have talked about the importance of challenges in human growth and development, and this importance is more than just skin deep. Our very bones must experience just the right amount of stress to grow correctly, and we must all experience stress in some form or another to continue our existence. Stress is a necessary aspect of life that knows no difference in class, religion, race, or diagnosis. And, when we are willing to identify with each other, to say, "Yes, I am different like you are also different," we realize that we all have special needs. We come to realize that we all have needs that must be acknowledged and accommodated at some point in our lives. Perhaps we are not as different from others as we may have originally thought. Seeing ourselves in others, despite apparent differences, humanizes us by acknowledging our diverse needs.

Humans, by nature, are driven to rank and categorize our world to make sense of the confusion we see around us. We tend to lift some people on a pedestal so high that we cannot reach them, while we trample others beneath our feet, relegating them to the muck and mire of human refuse. Neither of these extremes leads to relationships that bring true belonging and acceptance, and changing the words we use will only change the outward dressings.

To see genuine acceptance and true belonging, we must invest instead in eye-to-eye relationships. These are the only kind of relationships that can allow people to meet on equal, if albeit different, footing.

Chapter 3

Towards a Philosophy of Education

"Children are born persons."
- Charlotte Mason

My favorite educational philosopher is Charlotte Mason. She was a British educator in the late 19th and early 20th centuries and was a contemporary of the Italian educational philosopher Maria Montessori and the Austrian educational philosopher Rudolf Steiner. All three were influenced by great thinkers of the Romanticism and Transcendentalist periods, like Johann Wolfgang von Goethe, Friedrich Nietzsche, Ralph Waldo Emerson, Henry David Thoreau, and Georg Wilhelm Friedrich Hegel, just to name a few.

Were we to ask Mason, Montessori, and Steiner what they thought of each other's philosophies, they may not have admitted that their philosophies have anything in common. But more than 100 years later, I see so many similarities between them; certainly more than I see between them and our current system of education. However, Charlotte Mason remains my favorite.

There are many reasons I love Mason's philosophy. Perhaps a small part of it is Mason's connection to Louisa May Alcott. I loved reading Alcott's books as a child. I had every single book of hers that I could find in print at the time, but the *Little Women* trilogy was always my favorite, perhaps because so much of it was based on Louisa's own life and family. She had an unusual childhood growing up in Massachusetts and was educated by her father, Bronson Alcott, an educational philosopher in his own right. Louisa was surrounded by her father's friends which included Ralph Waldo Emerson and Henry David Thoreau. You see these influences throughout *Little Women*, including references to literature popular in Transcendentalist circles such as *The Pilgrim's Progress* by John Bunyan and writings by Goethe.

But you get even more insight into Bronson Alcott's educational philosophy from reading *Little Men*. Some people have wondered about the similarities between the school described in *Little Men* and the descriptions of Charlotte Mason's schools in England. As it turns out, Bronson Alcott took a trip to England to discuss educational philosophy with some of the people that Charlotte Mason later quotes in her books. So yes, I would say that *Little Men* is an apt description of a Charlotte Mason school.

As an avid fan of Transcendentalist authors like Louisa May Alcott, I cannot help but be drawn to Charlotte Mason's philosophy. But why do the educational ideas of Transcendentalism and Romanticism (including Charlotte Mason's philosophy) matter at all? Because balance matters.

German philosopher Georg Wilhelm Friedrich Hegel once tried to explain patterns of history in which societal views swing on a pendulum attempting to find balance in the extremes. As views became entrenched towards reason during the Enlightenment, there was a strong swing towards faith, giving rise to the Romanticism period. Either extreme, whether that of extreme reason or extreme faith, can be deadly. The swing towards extreme faith during certain historical periods caused persecution in the form of the Crusades, the Inquisition, and witch hunts. But, on the other hand, history has shown us that excessive reliance on reason has also led to persecution, exemplified by events like the Holocaust, eugenics, and racism.

As it turns out, Hegel theorized that both extremes are needed to find balance. Reason places value on what can be seen and measured, while faith places value on what is unseen and defies measurement. As Jane Austen put it, it is the balance between "sense and sensibility."

We are now living in a time when society as a whole leans toward reason. We measure how well children learn in school and then reward the teachers and schools that have the best scores. When we had a global health crisis, we insisted on only following "the science." But that is the interesting thing about reason and science. They only answer the specific questions you have asked, and as Charlotte Mason said,

> We teach children, too, not to 'lean (too confidently) to their own understanding'; because the function of Reason is to give logical demonstration
> (a) of mathematical truth,
> (b) of an initial idea, accepted by the will.
>
> In the former case, Reason is, practically, an infallible guide, but in the latter, it is not always a safe one; for, whether that idea be right or wrong, Reason will confirm it by irrefragable proofs.

Charlotte Mason wrote her magnum opus, *Towards a Philosophy of Education*, right after World War I, which allowed her, as an educator, to observe the events that led up to the war. She observed and criticized Germany's educational system at the time:

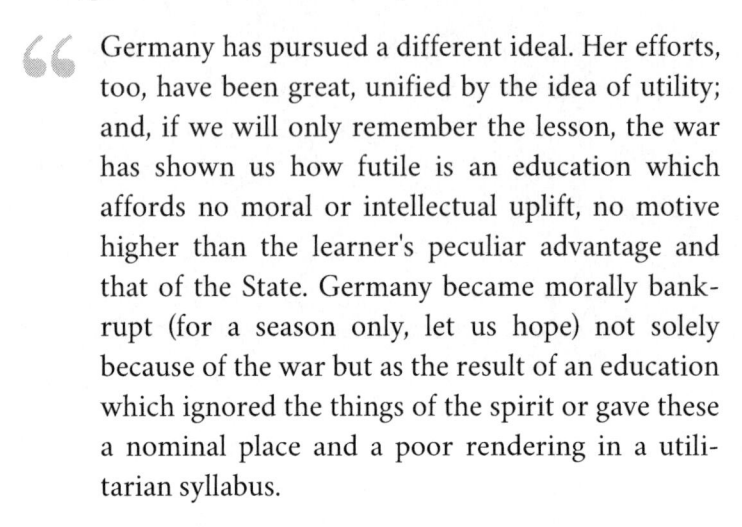

> Germany has pursued a different ideal. Her efforts, too, have been great, unified by the idea of utility; and, if we will only remember the lesson, the war has shown us how futile is an education which affords no moral or intellectual uplift, no motive higher than the learner's peculiar advantage and that of the State. Germany became morally bankrupt (for a season only, let us hope) not solely because of the war but as the result of an education which ignored the things of the spirit or gave these a nominal place and a poor rendering in a utilitarian syllabus.

A utilitarian education is not only futile as Mason suggests, but is also potentially dangerous. Leading up to World War I, Germany, like many other countries at the time, and not unlike us today, emphasized the importance of an education based on measurable and observable goals. However, their actions went to such an extent that a person's value was determined solely by those quantifiable objectives. This meant that there was no need to have any respect for individual countries (as in World War I) or individual people who did not meet the criteria for excellence (as in World War II).

How often do we consider the effects of our educational systems and what they might lead to? Not often enough, as Charlotte Mason is wont to point out:

> The educational thought we hear most about is, as I have said, based on sundry Darwinian axioms out of which we get the notion that nothing matters but physical fitness and vocational training. However important these are, they are not the chief thing. A century ago when Prussia was shipwrecked in the Napoleonic wars it was discovered

that not Napoleon but Ignorance was the formidable national enemy; a few philosophers took the matter in hand, and history, poetry, philosophy, proved the salvation of a ruined nation, because such studies make for the development of personality, public spirit, initiative, the qualities of which the State was in need, and which most advance individual happiness and success. On the other hand, the period when Germany made her school curriculum utilitarian marks the beginning of her moral downfall. History repeats itself.

Once again, we see history repeating itself. The Prussian model of utilitarian education eventually became the educational model for the United States, the United Kingdom, Germany, Japan, and others by the mid-nineteenth century. These countries were impressed by the possibilities of a mandatory compulsory education system for inspiring a nationalistic spirit. However, these same attributes eventually made way for the Nazi educational system. After Hitler outlawed homeschooling, it was easy for him to simply incorporate his own mandates into the national curriculum, which he did with great success. Despite many efforts to remove it, the only law that remains on the books in Germany from when Hitler was in power is the ban on homeschooling.

In the United States post-COVID, we have seen more than a 100% increase in the number of homeschooled students. I suspect this increase is a vote by the American people against a utilitarian model of education, which focuses the majority of instructional time on reading, writing, math, and many facts, regardless of whether that instruction is effective or not. But what good is an education rich in knowledge without the character development with which to use that knowledge wisely?

And which subjects are the first to be cut from school curricula? The liberal arts subjects are always the first to go because they do not serve an observable and measurable purpose.

Once again, we come across this phrase: "observable and measurable." The real question we must ask ourselves when contemplating a philosophy of education is, "What is the measure of a man?"

"The Measure of a Man" also happens to be the title of the highest viewer-ranked episode of *Star Trek: The Next Generation*. In this episode, the United Federation of Planets wants to re-assign the android named Data as if he were a piece of property belonging to the Federation. With his shipmates' help, Data fights for the right to choose his own destiny, and after a challenging case, the judge makes the following closing remarks:

> It sits there looking at me, and I don't know what it is. This case has dealt with metaphysics, with questions best left to saints and philosophers. I am neither competent nor qualified to answer those. I've got to make a ruling, to try to speak to the future. Is Data a machine? Yes. Is he the property of Starfleet? No. We have all been dancing around the basic issue. Does Data have a soul? I don't know that he has. I don't know that I have! But I have got to give him the freedom to explore that question himself. It is the ruling of this court that Lieutenant Commander Data has the freedom to choose.

And that is the question we are dancing around regarding education: Is a child a whole person? Or is he an empty jug waiting to be filled, or a computer to be programmed? The truth is that there is no way to prove either point. It falls within the realm of faith. The best thing we can do is to ask the question, what does it mean to be a person? Further, we must give children, and ourselves, the freedom to explore that question.

Charlotte Mason summed up her philosophy of education in just 20 principles, the first of which is "Children are born persons."

I have yet to find another educational philosophy that starts with the idea that children are whole persons. I suppose most people think this idea is too basic of a place to begin. However, the more I read and study educational philosophy, the more I become convinced that it is *the* most important place to start.

Nazi Germany did not see children as whole persons. They saw children only for the physical and mental value they could bring to the State. Those who were deemed to be physically or mentally inferior were terminated. And this idea continues even today. Recently, Iceland has come under scrutiny from the United Nations for a nearly 100% rate of terminating pregnancies with a prenatal diagnosis of Down syndrome.[1]

"Children are born persons" was relevant in Charlotte Mason's time and continues to be so today. Who we are as people, and therefore as a society, is determined by how we treat those most vulnerable.

Charlotte Mason's 20 Principles in Plain English

I took it upon myself to modernize Charlotte Mason's 20 Principles by looking at each principle through a neurodivergent lens (or you can reference Mason's original wording at the back of this book).

PRINCIPLE #1: Children are full people and should be accorded the same respect we afford adults.

PRINCIPLE #2: All children have potential.

PRINCIPLE #3: We all have rules we must obey in order to live with others, BUT

PRINCIPLE #4: Those rules are limited by our respect for

others as full persons, and we may not manipulate them in any way, whether by fear, love, suggestion, influence, or natural desire.

PRINCIPLE #5: Therefore, we have three educational instruments. Education is an *atmosphere*, a *discipline*, and a *life*.

PRINCIPLE #6: *Education is an atmosphere:* Children are most influenced by the atmosphere we provide. Who we are as people will have the most powerful impact on them rather than the activities and opportunities we provide them.

PRINCIPLE #7: *Education is a discipline:* We mindfully develop habits to help us achieve the things we want so we do not constantly have to think about every single decision.

PRINCIPLE #8: *Education is a life:* We are people: body, mind, and soul. We all need regular and balanced sustenance to continue to grow and remain healthy.

PRINCIPLE #9: Children are not computers to be programmed but rather whole persons whose minds need to not merely learn about facts and ideas but truly digest those ideas.

PRINCIPLE #10: As such, a child's only true teacher is themselves because they are the only one who can digest the various ideas presented to them. Anything less would be indoctrination.

PRINCIPLE #11: Once a child has developed his sensory and language neural pathways to a point that learning can take place through the use of language, his curriculum should be generous and take care that facts are not presented without their informing ideas because –

PRINCIPLE #12: "Education is the Science of Relations" = it is the connections we make between a wide range of subjects and ideas that are the true work of education. Therefore, a child should receive a wide curriculum full of physical exercises, nature lore, handicrafts, science, art, and many living books. It is not our job to teach him all about anything but to help him find threads that connect our world.

PRINCIPLE #13: In creating a curriculum, three points must be considered:

1. He requires much knowledge to sustain his mind.
2. The knowledge should be varied so the diet his mind feeds upon will be well balanced.
3. Knowledge should be communicated through language appropriate to him because that is the way in which ideas are shared.

PRINCIPLE #14: We have not truly gained knowledge until we have digested those ideas and reproduced our understanding of those ideas. This is why conversations with our children are so important.

PRINCIPLE #15: We do not need to insult our children's intelligence by re-reading, summarizing, and questioning them to ensure their understanding. Present the material and allow them to make the connections that are there for them to make at that moment. No person's connections are better than those of another person's connections. They have been given a unique perspective with which to understand the world and that perspective is valid.

PRINCIPLE #16: We have two tools we can offer children as guidance: *the way of the will* and *the way of reason*.

PRINCIPLE #17: *The way of the will*: Children should be taught:

- There are the things we want and there are the things we choose (or will).
- Sometimes when we have difficulty doing something we know we should do, distracting ourselves with

something quite different can help us gather strength to return to a difficult task.
- It is often something entertaining or interesting that can be the best tool in turning our thoughts.
- With a little rest, we can return to the task with more energy, and it is by this experience that we learn how to self-regulate ourselves.

PRINCIPLE #18: *The way of reason*: We teach children not to become too trusting of the scientific reasoning of the day because reason only (a) proves a mathematical proof or (b) creates arguments to back up any idea whether right or wrong.

PRINCIPLE #19: As children become mature enough to understand, they must be taught that their most important job is not to ask "Can we?" but "Should we?" To help them, we provide them with guiding principles and a wide range of ideas so that their choices are not based on a single perspective.

PRINCIPLE #20: Although much attention is paid to the development of a child's body and mind, we do not neglect the feeding of a child's soul – that part that is not the mind and not the body – because it is this that gives a person value, not how talented they are physically or mentally.

Chapter 4

Towards a Psychology of Being

"The science of psychology has been far more successful on the negative than on the positive side... It has revealed to us much about man's shortcomings, his illnesses, his sins, but little about his potentialities, his virtues, his achievable aspirations, or his psychological health."
- Abraham Maslow

We will come back to Charlotte Mason and her educational philosophy later. Now I would like to introduce you to my favorite psychological philosopher, Abraham Maslow, who was born about fifteen years before Charlotte Mason died. For those aware of my professional background, Abraham Maslow might seem like an odd choice.

I received my training as a School Psychologist from a program steeped in the Behaviorist school of thought. Behaviorism, made famous by Ivan Pavlov and his dogs, focuses strictly on that which can be observed objectively and looks for patterns in behavior. Unfortunately, this emphasis on the physically observable tends to view people as "empty slates." Behaviorists can unintentionally risk treating their clients like lab rats if they do not have a strong balance of respect for personhood. This is one reason that Applied Behavior Analysis (ABA) has come under fire in recent years.

And because I was interested in brain development, I also chose an emphasis in Neuropsychology, which falls into the Cognitive school of thought. Cognitive psychologists work to understand how people think, learn, perceive, and remember. Due to the complexity of the brain, Cognitive psychology touches on quite a few other disciplines, such as neuroscience, linguistics, psychiatry, and even psychoanalysis. Yes, I said psychoanalysis, as in Sigmund Freud. His ideas, like the "Oedipus Complex," have become significantly less in vogue since the Third Industrial Revolution opened so many doors in computer technology, neurobiology, and pharmacology. However, both psychoanalysis and Cognitive psychology focus on how the mind processes information.

Interestingly, a third school of thought in psychology is Humanism, and it has often been referred to as the "third force," opposing both Behaviorism and psychoanalysis. This is a pretty accurate description of Humanism. Humanists support the belief that humans, as individuals, are unique beings and should be recognized and treated as such. On the other hand, both Behavioral analysis and psychoanalysis strive to analyze what drives our behavior with the goal of changing or rehabilitating that behavior. But Humanism seeks to support people in achieving and fulfilling their potential or, put another way, becoming the best versions of themselves that they can be. Behaviorism and psychoanalysis were both born during the age of the Enlightenment, while Humanism, like Charlotte Mason, was born during the late Romanticism period. Abraham Maslow also belonged to the Humanist school of thought.

Maslow is most famous for his "Hierarchy of Needs" theory, but we'll discuss this in more depth later on in this chapter.

Maslow has received criticism for his lack of supporting scientific data, but I am always open to considering ideas even if there is currently no data to back them up. After all, science only answers the precise questions that we ask and if we don't ask the right questions, then we won't get the right answers.

Recently, he has come under fire again for possibly stealing ideas from the Siksika (Blackfoot) Nation, although that accusation turned out to be false. Members of the Siksika Nation investigated the accusation by going through Maslow's published work as well as his unpublished articles, journals, and other personal writings.[1] They discovered that Maslow revered their culture and was certainly influenced by it. However, like many influential relationships, that influence came together with Maslow's other past relationships and experiences to form a completely new perspective.

Maslow wanted to explore concepts that could help humans reach higher levels of functioning, possibly achieving 75% or even 100% of their potential. He called this "Self-Actualization." But the questions Maslow chose to ask, and how he ended up creating his hierarchy of needs, were shaped by his Western perspective with its emphasis on individuality. Conversely, the Siksika Nation emphasizes community support because they believe individuals are born self-actualized with a duty to assist in community development.

It might seem subtle, but that single foundational shift results in a cascade of differences. For example, in the Siksika Nation and other First Nations, a giveaway ceremony is held where tribe members give away valuable possessions. It is not the equivalent of donating your old and unwanted items to the local Goodwill store. To give things of value to others is seen as a sacred act within the Siksika society. And those who are the most generous are often seen as the wealthiest in the Siksika society.

The word *sacrifice* originally meant "something set apart" or "to make sacred." In fact, the word *poverty* is absent from the vocabulary of many First Nations due to their community-centered perspective. In the book *Decolonizing Wealth: Indigenous Wisdom to Heal Divides and Restore Balance* by Edgar Villanueva, the author records a story of Lakota Nation members being asked how they might translate the word *poverty*. The closest translation they could suggest was "someone without family." What a beautiful perspective to understand that our real wealth comes from our interconnectedness!

When Maslow witnessed the giveaway ceremony, he realized that 80-90% of people in the Siksika Nation met his self-esteem criteria. However, only 5-10% of people in his own culture met his criteria for self-esteem. Maslow then decided to conduct a more thorough investigation into the differences between his culture and the Siksika culture.

One area Maslow specifically looked at was how children were raised in both cultures. In the Siksika culture, children were raised permissively and treated as equal members of society. Even though Siksika children had a great deal of freedom, they still listened to their elders and participated in the community, even as young children. And isn't that a lovely idea for society to see babies as already self-actualized and worthy of being treated as full citizens? I, too often, hear children express sentiments like, "No one cares what I think. I'm just a kid." What kind of a difference might a shift in perspective like that make?

To experience self-actualizing moments, you must be your most authentic self. Otherwise, you are "other-actualizing" instead of self-actualizing. If we look at small pockets in our society, we can already identify some where children are allowed to be more authentic. Homeschoolers, for instance, have fewer societal expectations, mainly because their primary influences come from within the home. Shelby Dersa, author of *Homeschooling Wildflowers: Bring Your Child with Dyslexia, ADHD, Dysgraphia, or Dyscalculia Back to Their Natural Environment*, wrote, "Homeschoolers are not weird, they simply feel comfortable truly being themselves in a world where children feel pressured to be like their peers, and society confuses the two."

In Siksika culture, a person is considered self-actualized at birth and is expected to "listen within" to find their most authentic self. However, in Western culture, there is this tendency to view children as clay to be molded into our own ideal. Those few adults in Western culture that make a point of honoring the personhood of all individuals, no matter how small they might be, stand out as giants to children!

Fred Rogers continues to be revered by people of all ages globally, even decades after his passing, because of his respectful treatment of those individuals often marginalized by society. In a 1969 episode of his television show *Mister Rogers' Neighborhood*, he quietly confronted segregation when he sat with his feet in a kiddie pool with a black actor (playing the part of the beloved Officer Clemmons) during a time when swimming pools were segregated by race. To ensure that children with visual impairments could also enjoy his show, he began narrating his actions, like feeding the fish. And day after day, he would tell the children in his audience, "You've made this day a special day, by just your being you. There's no person in the whole world like you, and I like you just the way you are."

If we listen to the Siksika Nation as Abraham Maslow did, or if we listen to Fred Rogers, as millions of children did between 1968 and 2001, we learn that what is required for self-actualization is simply believing that we are, in fact, self-actualized. Eventually, the experiences that lead to immense leaps in individual growth will happen if we continue to be ourselves and look for the lessons around us.

So what is this Hierarchy of Needs, and how does it influence self-actualization? Abraham Maslow introduced his idea of a Hierarchy of Needs in a 1943 paper called "A Theory of Human Motivation," published in the journal *Psychological*

Review. In it, he theorized that humans have at least five basic needs:

1. Physiological
2. Safety
3. Love
4. Esteem
5. Self-Actualization

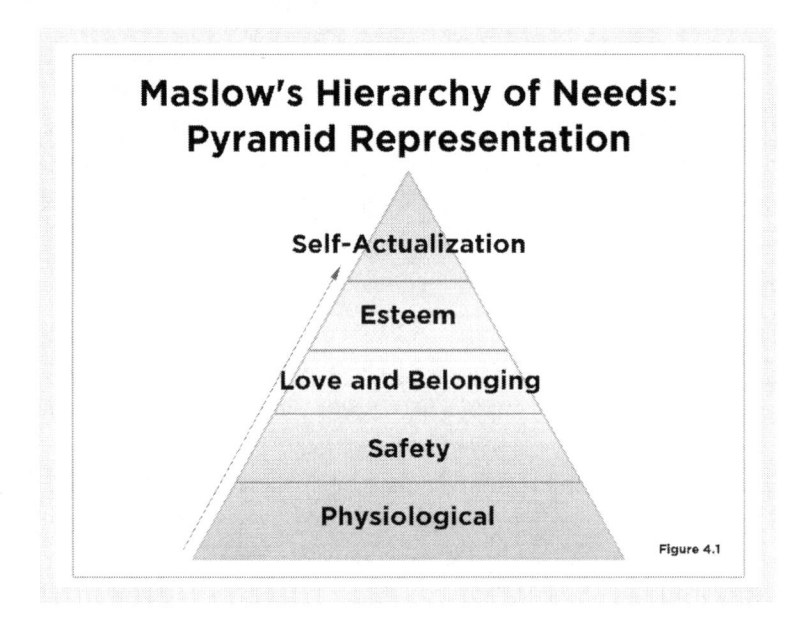

Maslow's Hierarchy of Needs: Pyramid Representation

- Self-Actualization
- Esteem
- Love and Belonging
- Safety
- Physiological

Figure 4.1

This is the image that most people are familiar with regarding Maslow's hierarchy of needs. But the pyramid image was actually first published in a *Journal of Business Horizons* article by Charles McDermid, "How Money Motivates Men,"[2] about 10 years before Abraham Maslow's death. But Maslow himself never represented his Hierarchy of Needs graphically. Further, professors Todd Bridgman, Stephen Cummings, and John Ballard, suggested that Maslow's theory is better understood as a ladder where individuals can be on multiple rungs at once.[3]

Before his death, Maslow expanded his theory to include at least eight basic needs:

1. Physiological
2. Safety
3. Love and Belonging
4. Esteem
5. Cognitive
6. Aesthetic
7. Self-Actualization
8. Transcendence.

(A detailed outline of Maslow's final version of his Hierarchy of Needs has been included at the end of this chapter.)

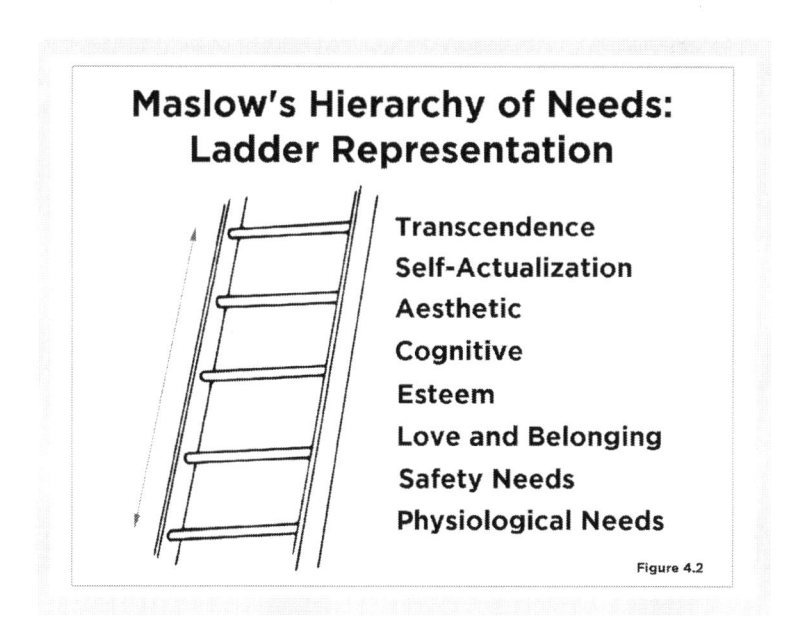

Maslow's Hierarchy of Needs: Ladder Representation

Transcendence
Self-Actualization
Aesthetic
Cognitive
Esteem
Love and Belonging
Safety Needs
Physiological Needs

Figure 4.2

The ideas of self-actualization and transcendence are universal. Charlotte Mason was indirectly influenced by Transcendentalist authors of her time, such as Ralph Waldo Emerson and Henry David Thoreau. Emerson, in turn, was greatly inspired by the Bhagavad Gita and played a significant role in introducing yoga philosophy to the West for the first time. Additionally, Transcendence is the eighth rung in both Maslow's hierarchy and Patanjali's *Yoga Sutras*.

In the 1994 movie *Little Women*, Jo March says to Professor Baer, "Well, my mother and father were part of a rather unusual circle in Concord. Do you know the word Transcendentalist?" To which Professor Baer responds, "But this is German Romantic philosophy! We throw off all of our constraints and come to know ourselves through insight and experience."

But what is transcendence? Vocabulary.com defines transcendence as:

> Transcendence comes from the Latin prefix trans-, meaning 'beyond,' and the word scandare, meaning 'to climb.' When you achieve transcendence, you have gone beyond ordinary limitations. The word is often used to describe a spiritual or religious state, or a condition of moving beyond physical needs and realities. One way to achieve transcendence spiritually might be to fast for a long time. If you have trouble letting go of material needs, then you will have a difficult time achieving transcendence.

This isn't a bad explanation, and similar concepts have been explored in popular movies like *The Matrix* and *Doctor Strange*.

But the best explanation I have found is the comparison to mycelium or fungus spores. The mycelium network located underneath a forest floor connects the entire ecosystem together and is often referred to as the "wood wide web."[4] If that forest is destroyed by fire, it is the mycelium network and its interconnectedness that gives rebirth to the ecosystem. You can see this when you observe a "fairy ring" or mushrooms growing in a ring-like formation. Transcendence is the idea that on the deepest level, we are all connected by a spark of the Divine, and when we tap into that, we transcend to something greater than our individual selves. This awareness humbles us by revealing our lack of omniscience, evokes gratitude for unearned blessings, and reinstates our relationships with each other and the universe.

Maslow's Hierarchy of Needs

(adapted from Simply Psychology[5])

1. **Physiological Needs:** biological requirements for human survival. If these needs are not satisfied, the human body cannot function optimally. Maslow considered physiological needs the most important. All other needs are secondary to physiological needs.
2. **Safety Needs:** the need to feel secure and safe: People want to experience order, predictability, and control in their lives, such as emotional security, financial security, law and order, social stability, property, health, and well-being, as well as freedom from fear.
3. **Love and Belonging Needs:** the need to feel that one is loved and belongs: Belonging refers to a human emotional need for interpersonal relationships, affiliating, connectedness, and being part of a group, such as friendship, trust, acceptance, receiving and giving affection, and love.
4. **Esteem Needs:** the need to feel valuable. Maslow classified esteem needs into two categories: esteem for oneself; desire for reputation or respect from

others. Maslow indicated that the need for respect is most important for children.
5. **Cognitive Needs:** the need for meaning and predictability. Maslow felt that humans have an innate need to grow both physically and mentally; to learn, explore, discover, and create to increase our understanding of the world around us.
6. **Aesthetic Needs:** the appreciation and search for beauty, balance, form, etc. Maslow recognized that while physical and mental growth is essential, so is refreshment in the form of experiencing beauty around us in all its forms.
7. **Self-actualization Needs:** the realization of personal potential. Maslow describes this as the desire to live up to one's potential.
8. **Transcendence Needs:** when a person becomes motivated by values that transcend beyond self. This is sometimes referred to as "Spiritual Needs" and implies that humans are not solely defined by their physical and mental aspects, but that they also possess a third aspect commonly referred to as the soul.

Chapter 5

The Power of Myth and Personal Transformation

"Mythology, in other words, is Psychology misread as Biography, History, and Cosmology."
- Joseph Campbell

Before we continue with Charlotte Mason's 20 Principles and Abraham Maslow's Hierarchy of Needs, I must introduce you to one more person: Joseph Campbell.

Campbell was born around the same time as Maslow and spent most of his professional career as a professor of Literature at Sarah Lawrence College in New York. He is one of the most impactful figures in contemporary Mythology discourse. He was also recognized for his work in comparative religion as he said, "Myth is what we call other people's religion."

Universal themes abound in both religion and mythology. Campbell is perhaps most well-known by the general public (and most infamously known by academics) for his theory of the monomyth, the idea that all myths follow the same basic pattern. He theorized that the monomyth indicated a subconscious yearning for meaning and connection that is shared by all human beings, regardless of cultural or geographical boundaries. The most complete explanation of his monomyth theory can be found in his book *The Hero with a Thousand Faces*.

Mythology is the way we have historically wrestled with the larger questions of life: who we are, our place in the universe, and our purpose. Mythology and its universal themes can be seen in references from classic literature to pop culture. The same stories are told over and over again in different ways, which supports Campbell's idea that we all yearn for meaning and connection.

Take Star Wars, for instance, as an example. George Lucas, creator of the *Star Wars* movie series, has repeatedly stated that his inspiration for the series came from Campbell's book. But the connection between Campbell and Lucas goes deeper.

Joseph Campbell had a keen interest in Indian Mythology and delved into studying Sanskrit, a language that George Lucas had some exposure to during his stay in India with The Beatles under Maharishi Mahesh Yogi. In fact, Lucas' time in India made such an impression on him that it influenced the themes he used in *Star Wars*. He even modeled the character of Yoda after the Maharishi to share the same mannerisms and speech cadence.[1]

Campbell and Lucas were later introduced by a mutual friend and became fast friends, likely due to their common interests. Campbell later visited Lucas at the Skywalker Ranch to watch the *Star Wars* movies. Additionally, they filmed an interview with Bill Moyers called *The Power of Myth*, discussing Campbell's monomyth and its impact on Star Wars. However, *Star Wars* is just one of many films influenced by Campbell's work in Mythology.

The creation of *The Lion King* was greatly influenced by a Disney Studios internal office memo titled *A Practical Guide to the Hero with a Thousand Faces* written by story consultant Chris

The Power of Myth and Personal Transformation

Vogler. In his seven-page memo, Vogler summarized Campbell's Hero's Journey into twelve steps:

1. The Ordinary World
2. The Call of Adventure
3. Refusal of the Call
4. Meeting the Mentor
5. Crossing the First Threshold
6. Tests, Allies, Enemies
7. Approach the Innermost Cave
8. The Ordeal
9. Reward
10. The Road Back
11. Resurrection
12. Return with the Elixir

(For your convenience, the 12 steps with complete descriptions have been included at the end of this chapter.)

Whether Campbell's theory of the monomyth influenced Disney Studios or it just happened to align with the original guiding vision of Walt Disney, the Hero's Journey is present in a long list of Disney films both before and after the office memo. You can see a hero journeying through each of the twelve steps in films such as *The Sword and the Stone, Snow White, Cinderella, Peter Pan, Pinocchio, Sleeping Beauty, Beauty and the Beast, Aladdin, Pocahontas, Brave, Mulan, Up, ET: Extra-Terrestrial, Oh Brother Where Art Thou, Braveheart,* and *Zorro* to name just a few.

In addition to Lucasfilm and Disney Studios, Campbell's work on Mythology has also influenced others, such as Richard Adams and his book *Watership Down* and Dan Brown, author of *The DaVinci Code,* who modeled his Robert Langdon character after Campbell himself.

In a documentary called *The Hero's Journey in Film,* Ciaran Michael Vejby identified more than 90 films that included the adventure, struggle, redemption, and victory of the Hero's Journey. Some of these include classic film series like *The Matrix, Indiana Jones, Men in Black, Batman, The Hunger Games, The Lord of the Rings, Harry Potter, How to Train Your Dragon, Star Trek, Batman,* and *Superman.*

Vejby also includes *Spiderman,* but none of the other Marvel story arcs created by Stan Lee made the list. The Marvel Universe is the creation of Stan Lee, the oldest son of Jewish immigrants. According to the book *Stan Lee: A Life in Comics* by Liel Leibovitz, Lee's Jewish background heavily influenced his creation of the Marvel universe, which includes several prominent and openly Jewish characters. However, Campbell's understanding of Jewish mythos is lacking for someone who claims to have such a thorough knowledge of world mythology. To the point, he appears to treat Christian mythos and Jewish mythos as if cut from the same cloth, which it is not. Judaism is far more Eastern in thought, and while this is a widespread misconception, it causes me to question what Campbell has to say about the mythos of other Eastern cultures.

Some academics argue that Campbell's theory of the monomyth is too superficial and his understanding of Eastern Mythology, specifically Indian mythology, is, at best, overstated. Campbell's monomyth theory has another problem though, as I've discovered through reading his writings. In the book *People Love Dead Jews,* author Dara Horn points out that literature doesn't always adhere to the same pattern:

> I began to see that the major works in these Jewish languages almost never involved characters getting saved, or having epiphanies, or experiencing moments of grace. In fact, as I read my way through foundational works in these literatures, I saw that many of the canonical stories and novels

in modern Yiddish and Hebrew literature actually didn't have endings at all.

Horn says that, much like the Jewish Bible with its relatively dry final passages of Chronicles, Jewish literature also often just suddenly ends. And in Sholem Aleichem's *Tevye the Dairyman*, which was the basis for the Broadway play *Fiddler on the Roof*,

> Tevye himself never changes. He never learns anything; he never realizes anything; he never has an epiphany or a moment of grace. And he's certainly never rescued or saved. Instead he just keeps enduring, which feels achingly realistic.

It turns out that "many of our expectations of literature are based on Christianity – and not just Christianity, but the precise points at which Christianity and Judaism diverge" (Horn). Perhaps not all cultures' literature fit the twelve bullet points of the Hero's Journey due to its Western-centric values.

But Campbell is not just an academic mythologist. For all of his complications, Campbell was a lifelong student of the liberal arts. He embraced the humanities and saw myth as a form of expression across cultures in all forms of art. Campbell was influenced by many artists and writers of the Romantic period including Maslow, Nietzsche, Carl Jung, and James Joyce.

Campbell knew that mythology is most valuable when it represents human expression through art, whether in the form of oral narratives, literature, visual arts, dance, theater, or music. Art, at its core, is the retelling of a story through different lenses.

Campbell was an avid fan of both art and dance. He married dancer and choreographer Jean Erdman, who was also influenced by artists and writers of the Romantic period including the creators of Modern Dance, Isadora Duncan and Martha

Graham. (Fun fact: Duncan and Graham's work later inspired the Grecian Urn number in *The Music Man*).

Duncan and Graham, in turn, were greatly influenced by Nietzsche, who was interested in how art can be involved in the process of transformation. For Nietzsche, life's ultimate question was "Does it dance?"

Author Kimerer L. LaMothe, who wrote *Nietzsche's Dancers: Isadora Duncan, Martha Graham, and the Revaluation of Christian Values*, states:

> Nietzsche's ubiquitous references to dance are ever-present reminders that the work of overcoming oneself – of freeing oneself enough from anger, bitterness and despair to say 'Yes!' to life – is not just an intellectual or scientific task. An ability to affirm life demands bodily practices that discipline our minds to elemental rhythms, to the creativity of our senses, and to the 'great reason', our body, 'that does not *say* "I" but *does* 'I'.' Only when we engage in such practices will we have the sensory awareness we need in order to discern whether the values we create and the movements we make express love for ourselves and the Earth.

Perhaps, it is seeing art and its expression of myth as a way of understanding our past, present, and future that resonates with us so much.

Mythology, Psychology, and Theology are the study of who we are – not who we are individually but who we are collectively. For this reason, ancient peoples took greater care to preserve their stories than they did their technology or even their history. After all, it is our stories that best capture our ideas and understanding of not only who we are but who we wish to be when we and our progeny are long gone.

Joseph Campbell was a rather complicated man with many different facets, some of which may seem contradictory, but he understood that the stories we tell and the many art forms we use to tell those stories serve as the roadmap to self-knowledge, transcendence, and wisdom.

The Hero Stages

from *A Practical Guide to The Hero with a Thousand Faces* by Chris Vogler

1. THE ORDINARY WORLD: The hero is introduced in his ordinary world. Most stories take place in a special world, a world that is new and alien to its hero. If you're going to tell a story about a fish out of his customary element, you first have to create a contrast by showing him in his mundane, ordinary world.
2. THE CALL TO ADVENTURE: The hero is presented with a problem, challenge, or adventure.
3. REFUSAL OF THE QUEST: The hero is reluctant at first. Often at this point, the hero balks at the threshold of adventure.
4. MEETING THE MENTOR: The hero is encouraged by the wise old man or woman. By this time, many stories will have introduced a Merlin-like character who is the hero's mentor. The mentor can only go so far with the hero. Eventually, the hero must face the unknown by himself. Sometimes the wise old man is required to give the hero a swift kick in the pants to get the adventure going.
5. CROSSING THE THRESHOLD: The hero passes the first threshold and fully enters the special world of his story for the first time. This is the moment at

which the story takes off and the adventure gets going.
6. TESTS, ALLIES, AND ENEMIES: The hero encounters tests and helpers. The hero is forced to make allies and enemies in the special world and to pass certain tests and challenges that are part of his training.
7. THE INNERMOST CAVE/THE APPROACH: The hero reaches the innermost cave. The hero comes at last to a dangerous place, often deep underground, where the object of his quest is hidden.
8. THE SUPREME ORDEAL: The hero endures the supreme ordeal. This is the moment at which the hero touches bottom. He faces the possibility of death, brought to brink in a fight with a mythical beast. This is a critical moment in any story, an ordeal in which the hero appears to die and is born again. It's a major source of the magic of the hero myth. What happens is that the audience has been led to identify with the hero. We are encouraged to experience the brink-of-death feeling with the hero. We are temporarily depressed, then we are revived by the hero's return from death. You're never more alive than when you think you're going to die.
9. THE HERO SEIZES THE SWORD: Having survived death, beaten the dragon, slain the Minotaur, the hero now takes possession of the treasure he's come seeking. Sometimes the "sword" is knowledge and experience that leads to greater understanding and a reconciliation with hostile forces. The hero may also be reconciled with a woman. Women in these stories (or men if the hero is female) tend to be "shape-shifters." They appear to change in form or age, reflecting the confusing and constantly changing

aspects of the opposite sex as seen from the hero's point of view.
10. THE ROAD BACK: The hero's not out of the woods yet. Some of the best chase scenes come at this point, as the hero is pursued by the vengeful forces from whom he has stolen the elixir or the treasure.
11. THE RESURRECTION: The hero emerges from the special world, transformed by his experience.
12. RETURN WITH THE ELIXIR: The hero comes back to his ordinary world, but his adventure would be meaningless unless he brought back the elixir, or treasure, or some lesson from the special world. Sometimes it's just knowledge or experience, but unless he comes back with something, he's doomed to repeat the adventure until he does.

Chapter 6

The Power of a Story

"The purpose of a storyteller is not to tell you how to think, but to give you questions to think upon."
- Brandon Sanderson

We have talked now about 3 different individuals: Charlotte Mason, Abraham Maslow, and Joseph Campbell, and each one represents a sphere of influence over a specific area of my experience respectively: Homeschool Parent of Autistic Children, School Psychologist turned Private Consultant, and Autistic person with a special interest in mythology. (Honestly, you are lucky that I only spent one chapter talking about mythology!) These three individuals and their ideas represent the foundation of my personal and professional philosophy.

We spent the entire first half of the book dancing around the fundamental question: Who has value? Or put another way: Who is a whole person? And why does this matter? It matters because the rest of this book will focus on supporting children in becoming, self-actualizing, and transcending.

Who or what is capable of transcendence? Is it just certain

people? Or are all living things innately capable of transcendence? How do we define life? And who gets to define that? These are the questions that have "tried men's souls" for centuries.

Throughout history, people have come up with many different answers. Most infamously, the Nazis defined a whole person as Aryan, or those being of German or related descent. But even within the Nazis' definition, homosexuals and people with disabilities were not considered Aryan even if they were born to Aryan parents.

Sadly we often think that the dehumanization of people during World War II was limited to the Nazis, but it wasn't. As Dara Horn quotes in *People Love Dead Jews*, "We live on two myths - that we didn't know, and that we couldn't do anything even if we did know. This is the religion, and it isn't true. We knew plenty and could have done a lot."

But, Americans did more than ignore the plight of others. We also dehumanized the Japanese. Allied soldiers used the bones of fallen Japanese soldiers to make pen holders and letter openers as souvenirs.

Were these the only instances of dehumanization during World War II? Absolutely not! According to David Livingston Smith, author of the book *Less Than Human: Why We Demean, Enslave, and Exterminate Others*, each side in the conflict used propaganda to dehumanize the enemy so that their soldiers could easily and eagerly kill other human beings without guilt or remorse. How else could human beings be convinced to kill other human beings? The only answer was dehumanization.

A prime example of dehumanization based on race was the American system of chattel slavery from the 17th century through the 19th century. And this dehumanizing of people based on skin color did not end there. Even towards the end of the 20th century, lynchings were still commonplace, and those lynchings were not simple hangings. They were designed to torture and mutilate their victims and to invoke fear in others. No wonder we still collectively carry the trauma of this dehumanization.

The United States government also dehumanized Native Americans. Due to government policies, Native Americans slowly lost their lands, their traditions, and cultures. Finally, the U.S. government imprisoned them on reservations in 1851. The government then forcibly removed Native American children from their families and sent them to re-education "boarding" schools to "civilize the savage."[1] Children at these schools were often abused for speaking their native tongue or practicing their native culture. This practice wasn't outlawed until 1978.

Consider the consequences of these two instances of dehumanization based on race: the loss of language, culture, family, a sense of safety, the opportunity to grow up in a family instead of in slavery or a boarding school, and to learn how to be a parent. Those are all significant cultural losses that take generations to begin to heal. Let's not overlook the effort required to heal the emotional scars of belonging to a dehumanized lineage. And then there is the difficult shift in perspective needed to recognize that other people do not get to define your value.

These are just a few of the more well-documented instances of dehumanization. There are also instances of the dehumanization of immigrants that seem to have been forgotten in history. For example, Italian immigrants to America were not only ridiculed in drawings and songs but they were also subjected to physical attacks.

An article titled "Under Attack" from the Library of Congress[2] website states:

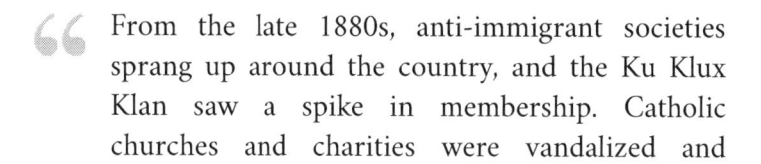

> From the late 1880s, anti-immigrant societies sprang up around the country, and the Ku Klux Klan saw a spike in membership. Catholic churches and charities were vandalized and

burned, and Italians attacked by mobs. In the 1890s alone, more than 20 Italians were lynched. One of the bloodiest episodes took place in New Orleans in 1891. When the chief of police was found shot to death on the street one night, the mayor blamed 'Sicilian gangsters' and rounded up more than 100 Sicilian Americans. Eventually, 19 were put on trial and, as the nation's Italian Americans watched nervously, were found not guilty for lack of evidence. Before they could be freed, however, a mob of 10,000 people, including many of New Orleans' most prominent citizens, broke into the jail. They dragged 11 Sicilians from their cells and lynched them, including two men jailed on other offenses. Italians worldwide were outraged, but the U.S. press generally approved of the action. It was the largest single mass lynching in U.S. history.

To combat these anti-Italian sentiments, Italian Americans popularized Christopher Columbus as an Italian American hero. It was Italian Americans' way of assimilating by finding a historically important Italian American.

And this is not the only instance of immigrants and their children working to find ways to endear themselves to their new country. Robert May, the author of *Rudolph the Red-Nosed Reindeer*, was born in the United States to Jewish immigrants. May often experienced ridicule for his stereotypical Jewish nose which caused him to be excluded by other children. When asked to write a Christmas story for Macy's Department Store, May drew on his own experiences to create Rudolph, a reindeer with an unusual nose who was often ridiculed and excluded. And as many Jewish Americans have found, there may not be a better way to endear yourself to Americans than writing a Christmas story or song. Approximately 75 Christmas songs have been written by Jewish Americans!

Then there are also those instances of dehumanization that include genocide, which is rather extensive, including Cambodian, Armenian, Greek, Circassian, Assyrian, Serbian, Romani, Rwandan, and Darfurian, to name a few.

Dehumanization is also not limited to just modernity, sex, or age.

We have documentation at least as far back as the 4th century BCE to the Siege of Melos, arguably one of the earliest genocides recorded in history.

Although both men and women can be objectified and thus dehumanized, women have been seen as the legal property of men throughout much of history.

And the more vulnerable populations who cannot always speak for themselves are more likely to experience dehumanization, such as elderly individuals or young children. Up until a few short decades ago, we did not even give infants anesthesia during surgery because we thought they could not feel pain, which shows that we did not see them as whole persons.

And those of us with disabilities are also often not seen as whole persons either. More than 90% of people with developmental disabilities are sexually abused, with 49% of victims abused at least ten times.[3]

In summary, no one is immune to dehumanizing or to being dehumanized by others. David Livingston Smith asked in *Less Than Human: Why We Demean, Enslave, and Exterminate Others*, why do we dehumanize others, and what can we do about it? He concludes that our propensity towards dehumanizing others comes from a combination of fear and using our reason to back up that fear.

As Master Yoda points out, "Fear is the path to the dark side. Fear leads to anger. Anger leads to hate. Hate leads to suffering."

We have a need to put things into categories to make sense

of the unorganized chaos of the world we find ourselves in. Even as young children, research shows that we group people by race out of a desire to identify those who are like us versus those who are not like us.

That said, I want to point out that Autistic children do not always do this, at least not in the same way. When I was a small child, I mistook a very dark-skinned man for my very pale-skinned father. I noticed he was tall and thin like my father but completely missed the significant difference in skin color. And it is not uncommon for Autistic children to take note of significantly different features than neurotypicals.

But all of us have this self-preserving tendency to categorize others in order to bring order and control to our world.

So what can we do to stave off the destruction we have seen throughout history, and especially within the last 500 years, thanks to this inherent need to categorize our world into black and white, Christian and Jew, Eastern and Western?

David Livingston Smith argues that we have 3 options: Science, Reason, and Feeling. But I don't see it this way. I think that we only have 2 options: Reason and Faith.

But what do these options mean? Science and Reason are really two sides of the same coin. While science often produces theories to test, it rarely produces laws that can be depended on in all circumstances. Meanwhile, Reason produces the same kind of product, but the tool used to test those theories is more often our own logic. And as we have come to recognize from the science of centuries past, what is "known" today will likely seem archaic and barbaric tomorrow.

Our methods for backing up our claims might have become more empirical over the ages, but they are still limited by the questions we ask, placing ourselves in the position of a god.

Like the people of old, building a tower to the heavens, we believe we have grown beyond the need for Faith or Feeling. But as poet Robert Browning wrote:

"I, Who want, am made for, and must have a God"

We cannot place ourselves in a god-like position. We must have something above us, whether you call that a god or not, to give us a sense of humility and to keep us from becoming too arrogant regarding our own greatness. Not doing so will only lead to a grievous end, as exemplified by the many examples in this book already.

But what of Feeling or Faith? Some might feel these words appear like entirely different things, but they share a similar foundation: Mythology.

While David Livingston Smith admits that using stories to engage feelings can be highly effective, he also points out that they can be equally effective for humanizing and dehumanizing people. So the question remains: if Mythology is so powerful, how do you pick the correct myths? The answer is you can't.

Just like we cannot place ourselves in a god-like position for Reason, we cannot put ourselves in a god-like position regarding choosing the correct stories. As author Robin Sharma said in his book *The Monk Who Sold His Ferrari*:

> *The Mind is an Excellent Servant, but a Terrible Master.*

Instead, what we can do is become lifelong students of stories. As we read widely, mixing together the wisdom of the ages, we will see some ideas repeated over and over again throughout the ages. This persistent wisdom clumps together to enforce a larger ideal, which we can then scoop out to help move us along the path toward wisdom and transcendence.

And remember, our best ideas tend to come when society has achieved a near-perfect balance between Faith and Reason. After all, the unique mixture of the Enlightenment and the

Great Awakening led to some very high ideals. High ideals that we still struggle to live up to today such as:

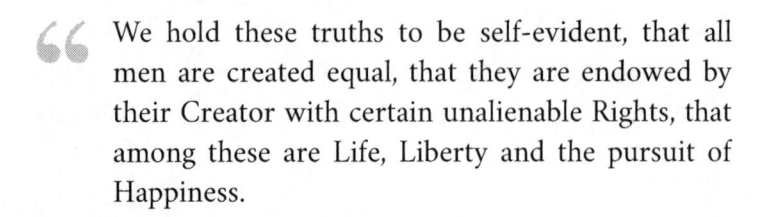

> We hold these truths to be self-evident, that all men are created equal, that they are endowed by their Creator with certain unalienable Rights, that among these are Life, Liberty and the pursuit of Happiness.

But just because we struggle to live up to them does not mean that they aren't valuable for spurring us on towards loftier aspirations.

Chapter 7

The Humanities: A Roadmap to Inner Peace

"Many young people suffer from a fear of the self. They do not feel at home in their own selves. The inner life is a place of dereliction, a no man's land, inconsolate, weird. The self has become a place from which to flee."

- Abraham Joshua Heschel

When I go to a homeschool convention, parents often ask me why they see so much "Charlotte Mason stuff," and the answer I give them is that people are thirsty for an education rich in the humanities.

Likely, if you are reading this book, you probably did not grow up with an education rich in the humanities, and you may not even know what that means. As the University of Illinois put it so eloquently, the humanities include a group of subjects focused on

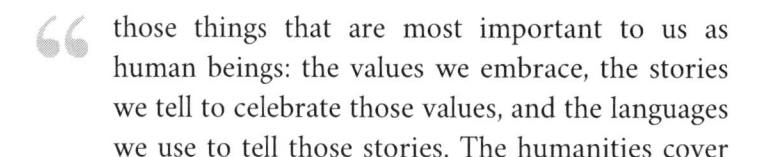

> those things that are most important to us as human beings: the values we embrace, the stories we tell to celebrate those values, and the languages we use to tell those stories. The humanities cover

the whole spectrum of human cultures across the entire span of human history.

It includes mythology, literature, religion, art, music, dance, theater, ancient and modern languages, history, philosophy, etc. It is the study of who we have been, who we are, and who we are becoming.

We can teach children all the facts and academic skills in the world. Still, without a grounding in the humanities, we can turn out little dictators. The humanities help us develop the wisdom to use that knowledge wisely. In a world where we have experienced so much scientific advancement in such a short time, where STEM and STEAM have reigned supreme, people subconsciously recognize a deep need and longing for the humanities, the cure for the anxiety and depression currently ravaging our society.

In a post-pandemic world where the prescription for anti-anxiety medications increased by 34%, emergency room visits for teenage suicide attempts increased by more than 50%, and almost all psychologists are too booked to accept new patients, it is not that we need better science. Rather we are starved for the humanities. For it is art, music, theater, poetry, and stories that act as a balm to our soul in times of trouble. And as we study the history and things left behind by our ancestors, we learn to dance on the tightrope of life with all its troubles and uncertainties.

Before we head into the practical application section of this book, I want to share with you some ideas from a mythos that are particularly meaningful to me. As I have studied myths from all over the world (remember, this is my special interest), I have come to see the stark philosophical difference in perspective between the East and West and how it often prevents us from communicating effectively. And the deeper I looked into the beliefs and writings of different cultures, the more I realized that, in many ways, Judaism uniquely straddles that divide between East and West and can serve as a bridge from one to the other. As such, I would like to present some specific ideas using Jewish philosophy that may help direct our thoughts as we move forward into how we can support our children's "becoming."

A popular but dry area of philosophical debate includes the "mind-body problem" popularized by Rene Descartes. The argument is whether the mind and brain are separate (also known as Dualism, favored primarily in the West) or completely entwined to the point of being one and the same (known as Monism, favored primarily in the East).

Generally speaking, monism has received the most support from the East and some prominent Jewish philosophers; however, in Jewish philosophy, monism is not a complete answer in itself. Yes, there is the entwined mind and body. But there is also, according to *Aish Magazine*, "In classical Jewish thinking, there is a Universal Consciousness that pervades the entire material world and beyond, as Isaiah wrote, 'the whole world is filled with His glory.'"

Or, put another way, the whole world is filled with a Universal Soul. And there you have the beginnings of body, mind, and soul, as first introduced in Jewish philosophy in Deuteronomy chapter 6, verse 5. The New King James Version translates it as follows, "You shall love the Lord your God with all your heart, with all your soul, and with all your strength."

However, I would like to look more closely at this line in its original Hebrew.

> וְאָהַבְתָּ אֵת יְהֹוָה אֱלֹהֶיךָ בְּכָל־לְבָבְךָ וּבְכָל־נַפְשְׁךָ וּבְכָל־מְאֹדֶךָ׃

> *v'ahav'ta et Adonai eloheykha b'kol l'vav'kha uv'kol nf'sh'kha uv'kol m'odekha*

Sometimes when translating Hebrew, we have to put the words in a different order for them to make sense in English, but in this case, the word order works perfectly in both languages. In "with all of your heart," b'kol l'vav'kha, the root word for heart is *lev*. In Hebrew, according to the *Jewish Virtual Library*,

> The interior of the body is conceived of as the seat of the inner life, of feeling and thought ... it is the lev that figures most often in references to the inner life, both emotional and – and this is its special sphere – intellectual.

In other words, b'kol l'vav'kha would best be translated as *with all your mind*.

Meanwhile, "with all your soul," uv'kol nef'sh'kha, the root word for soul, is *nefesh*. According to *Sefaria*:

> There are many words for the soul in Hebrew, but the most commonly used are nefesh and neshamah —both of which mean 'breath.' In truth, not just the human being, but also every created entity possesses a 'soul.' Animals have souls, as do plants and even inanimate objects; every blade of grass has a soul, and every grain of sand. Not only life, but also existence requires a soul to sustain it—a 'spark of G-dliness' that perpetually imbues its object with being and significance. A soul is not just the engine of life; it also embodies the why of a thing's existence, its meaning and purpose. It is a thing's "inner identity, its raison d'être. Just like the 'soul' of a musical composition is the composer's vision that energizes and gives life to the notes played in a musical composition—the actual notes

are like the body expressing the vision and feeling of the soul within them. Each soul is the expression of G-d's intent and vision in creating that particular being.

This is not unlike the writings of the ancient Yogis, with whom the ancient Jews had an ongoing relationship. Both see the breath as a connection between the mind-body and the soul. And both utilize the breath as a focal point in meditation. And finally, uv'kol m'odekha, "with all your strength," the root word translated as strength, is *me'od*.

These days, me'od has come to be used as an adverb like "very." However, in this unusual context where it appears by itself, which only happens one other time in all of the Tanakh, it is translated to mean "muchness" or "might." I want to suggest that we consider it to mean "matter," implying that it encompasses all of the physicality we have.

And there we have it, the first instance of the Jewish conception of the body, mind, and soul.

Of course, this is not the last time that we see this conception of the human being. We see this concept repeated again in the New Testament Gospel of Mark, chapter 12. We also see this in Plato's *Tripartite Model of the Soul*, which greatly influenced Christian writers such as Clement of Alexandria and Gregory of Nyssa.

And it is not just the West where we see these ideas. You also see a similar concept in the Bhagavad Gita using a chariot metaphor. The body is compared to a chariot pulled by horses representing the physical senses. The mind is the chariot's driver, which holds the reins and guides the body, and the soul is the master of the chariot, who sits beside the driver as the true observer. This concept subsequently influences the development of Yoga and Martial Arts as methods to strengthen the collective focus of body, mind, and soul. In later centuries, the Islamic philosopher, Mulla

Sadra, came to similar conclusions, and there has even been a Pyramid of Human Needs developed based on his work.

We have also seen this concept of body, mind, and soul repeated in Charlotte Mason's 20 Principles of Education and Abraham Maslow's Hierarchy of Needs.

Because of the widespread usage of body, mind, and soul, this is the concept I want to use as we move through the practicality of supporting children in becoming. While it may not be the most scientifically valid explanation, it is a way we have traditionally compartmentalized the different aspects of ourselves, even if our verbiage and interpretations vary somewhat between cultures.

You may wonder if I am attempting to promote the idea of moral relativism. No, just because two people have similar features does not mean they are the same person or even twins! I am advocating for a common vocabulary and framework.

As individuals, we all have different experiences that interact with our unique individuality producing a different perception of the world around us. I see each one of us as a gift to the world. I learn from the diverse individuals who cross my path every single day. Even if I disagree with them, they ignite questions and ideas that might not have crossed my mind otherwise, perhaps even ideas that I must wrestle with in my mind but which will potentially lead me towards a deeper understanding. They show me ways of viewing the world that would never have occurred to me otherwise.

Again, you may ask if I am insisting on a specific religious construct or any religious construct at all? No, you can view these thoughts through whatever ideology you call home.

Let me repeat: I am simply advocating for a common vocabulary and framework.

And if I honestly see each one of us as a gift to the world, then I must also respect the individuality of myself and others enough to not insist on sameness. Besides, wouldn't it be boring if every gift you received was always the same? It wouldn't make for a very interesting world, would it?

Finally, how do we define transcendence within this common vocabulary and framework?

Abraham Joshua Heschel was a Polish-American Rabbi who advocated for the civil rights of African Americans during the Civil Rights Movement. He called self-transcendence the act of moving from self-centeredness toward God-centeredness. Some might call this meditation. Heschel calls it prayer. In his essay "On Prayer," he says:

> All things have a home, the bird has a nest, the fox has a hole, the bee has a hive. A soul without prayer is a soul without a home. Weary, sobbing, the soul, after roaming through a world festered with aimlessness, falsehoods and absurdities, seeks a moment in which to gather up its scattered life, in which to divest itself of enforced pretensions and camouflage, in which to simplify complexities, in which to call for help without being a coward. Such a home is prayer. Continuity, permanence, intimacy, authenticity, earnestness are its attributes. For the soul, home is where prayer is. In his cottage, even the poorest man may bid defiance to misery and malice. That cottage may be frail, its roof may shake, the wind may blow through it, the storms may enter it, but there is where the soul expects to be understood. Just as the body, so is the soul in need of a home.

He also points out what many of us could also claim to be true today:

> Many young people suffer from a fear of the self. They do not feel at home in their own selves. The inner life is a place of dereliction, a no man's land, inconsolate, weird. The self has become a place from which to flee.

Far more significant than any developmental or academic needs, inner peace is our most profound, and often overlooked, need.

This book is a call to support young people in learning to feel at home in their own selves and to enjoy an inner life of peace.

Part Two

Practical Application

Chapter 8

Development: A Roadmap to Education

"Biology gives you a brain. Life turns it into a mind."
- Jeffrey Eugenides

In this section of the book, I'll explain my consultation process and how I determine the most effective approach for maximizing children's progress with minimal parental effort.

The first thing I do when working with a family is to give them a developmental rating scale designed to determine where the child is in their development. Determining where a child is developmentally is essential because development typically follows a general pattern. Determining where a child is developmentally can help us better understand what they might need help with to take the next step in cognitive development.

Much of our understanding of children's cognitive development comes from a Swiss Developmental Psychologist named Jean Piaget. His 1936 "Theory of Cognitive Development" determined that children's brains work differently than the brains of adults. Before this, people assumed that children weren't as intelligent as adults.

According to Piaget's "Four Stages of Development," the brain develops in stages, and certain types of information are developmentally inappropriate for children at different stages of development.

This makes logical sense, given what we have since learned about how the brain grows and develops: language tends to form in a particular order and comprises the same parts of speech regardless of the language learned. And we see definite patterns in other areas of learning as well. For example, it is well known that children generally do not develop a sense of chronology until about the age of seven. I say *generally* because we are continuing to expand our understanding of cognitive development, and only just recently have we been exploring a different modality of language development called Gestalt Language Processing.

Whether or not cognitive development can be easily divided up into four different stages as Piaget suggests is still up for debate; however, it is generally agreed that development does tend to follow a pattern, even if there are occasional exceptions.

However, one area that Piaget did not address was a child's culture and social environment. This line of thought was proposed at about the same time by Soviet Social Psychologist Leo Vygotsky through his concept of a "Zone of Proximal Development."

Vygotsky believed that a child's development was not nearly as important as the influence of what he called a "More Knowledgeable Other." Through social and cultural language-based interactions, this "More Knowledgeable Other," likely a parent or teacher, could provide appropriate scaffolding to make something accessible beyond the child's current level of development. Therefore, Vygotsky believed that the child's development and experiences were less important than the influence of "More Knowledgeable Others."

I have been rather surprised at how popular his ideas are

among some proponents of Charlotte Mason's philosophy of education because Vygotsky placed more emphasis and responsibility on the teacher than the child. In contrast, Charlotte Mason believed that all education must be self-education. However, I think that perhaps Vygotsky's untimely death at the age of thirty-seven, as well as his own cultural biases, may have prevented him from further developing his theories.

We see the torch of Vygotsky's work picked up again by Reuven Feuerstein, an Israeli Developmental Psychologist. Feuerstein's "Theory of Mediated Learning Experience" suggests that all learning can be divided into *direct learning* and *mediated learning*.

Mediated learning can be indispensable to a child's development because the mediator, or parent, can help the child develop prerequisite skills that make direct learning effective. Research has shown that hearing children of deaf parents cannot learn spoken language simply by passively watching television. It does appear that human facilitation of the environment is important in the development of pre-requisite skills that make direct learning possible.

Almost a century has passed since these men first began their work in cognitive development. Since then, we have learned much about the brain. However, all three men remain influential powerhouses in Educational Psychology, though not without criticism. Although Vygotsky and Feuerstein are often seen in opposition to Piaget, I find that placing the work of Vygotsky and Feuerstein within the developmental context of Jean Piaget's "Four Stages of Cognitive Development" allows us to not only identify where a child is in his development but also allows us to optimize his development and education.

Genetics can also impact development to a certain degree. And while we cannot change the genes a child is born with, we can provide environmental support to optimize the very best expression of those genes. We have to begin with figuring out where a child is developmentally. It is only then that we can determine what environmental supports will be the most effective.

According to Jean Piaget's theory, the "Four Stages of Cognitive Development" are:

1. Sensorimotor Stage
2. Preoperational Stage
3. Concrete Operational Stage
4. Formal Operational Stage

Let's look at each stage in more detail.

The Sensorimotor Stage

The Sensorimotor Stage usually occurs between the developmental ages of birth to two years. Notice I said both "usually" and "developmental ages." These are two critical distinctions. All persons are unique and never do everything at precisely the same time or in the same way. However, there are common trends in development, so this is what I mean by "usually." Second, the ages associated with Piaget's Stages are typical for these areas of development. In accordance with the research on Piaget's Stages, children with developmental delays also often experience delays in their advancement through Piaget's Stages.

The child's primary job in the Sensorimotor Stage is to develop and integrate their senses and motor functions. Children at this age spend most of their time learning to sit up, crawl, walk, run, and explore their world with their senses. As their senses and motor skills develop and integrate better, they become capable of more and more intentional behavior. However, their behavior is not entirely unintentional even as newborns.

In 1974, researchers created a pacifier that played different sounds to gauge a newborn's response to various stimuli, including the voice of the baby's mother. The researchers found that the infants consistently changed their sucking rate when they heard a familiar voice compared to an unfamiliar voice. So, even though newborns are not capable of showing intentional behavior in the same way that we as adults do, they can show intention with regard to the behaviors that they have within their developmental control. It takes time for a newborn to integrate their sensory and motor pathways for life outside the womb, just like it also takes time for us to re-integrate our sensory and motor pathways after a severe injury. By the end of this stage, they are beginning to exhibit more abstract problem-solving skills, such as using words or gestures to communicate and pretend. While Vygotsky's writings may not seem relevant here, all we have to do is look at neglected children's development to see just how important a child's environment is to his early development.

The Preoperational Stage

Most children are in the Preoperational Stage from two to seven years of age. We now know, thanks to neuroscience, that the brain typically experiences significant myelination at two and seven years of age. (As an aside, this is why doctors recommend that children drink whole milk until two years old. Fat is required for the myelination process; this was an easy way to ensure that small children got enough fat. It has nothing to do with calcium.) This is a stage of development with many significant neurological changes. And if you think about the difference between a two-year-old and a seven-year-old, I think you will agree! In this stage, much emphasis is still placed on concrete thought but we do see an increase in abstract thought. At the age of two, children begin with a somewhat egocentric view, but by age seven, they have developed a limited ability to take the perspective of others.

We have said that from the very beginning, children are influenced by their environment and relationships. However, at this point where language begins to develop, we see the very early signs of what Vygotsky wrote about the importance of relationships and language in development. This is also the approximate age at which Feuerstein began working with children. Their language skills are still quite fundamental at this stage, and children at this stage often struggle with understanding that two things can look different yet still be the same.

The Concrete Operational Stage

From seven until twelve years of age, children are generally considered to be in the Concrete Operational Stage of Cognitive Development. At this stage, children develop a sense of chronology and can easily take the perspectives of others. These are valuable skills when it comes to formal education. Thus, I think Charlotte Mason was correct in her thoughts that formal education should be held off until the age of six or seven.

This stage of development is also where Vygotsky's importance of relationships and language becomes significant. By this point, all basic language skills have either developed or are in the process of developing, both oral communication and written communication. And as Charlotte Mason said, "Education is the science of relations."

However, I would use caution when interpreting the writings of Vygotsky and Feuerstein. To assume that there must be a "More Knowledgeable Other" to scaffold a child's thoughts is to steal from that child the opportunity to self-educate. However, it would also be folly to assume that each man is an island without relationships to enlighten his education. The challenge is in supporting a child without stealing his ability to self-determinate his own destiny. And for adults, this is an especially difficult challenge as there is an imbalance of power in the relationship between adults and children.

Given some of the significant academic development at this stage, this is an excellent time to mention another later theory that has often been associated with Vygotsky's Zone of Proximal Development: the "Dual Coding" theory by Sadoski and Paivio which postulates that cognition cannot happen without mental representation. This means we must visualize in our minds in order to remember (and thus comprehend) new information and experiences. In layman's terms, memory is *typically* encoded visually. In other words, a picture is worth a thousand words and therefore takes up less processing space.

Sadoski and Paivio proposed that we have two separate visualization systems. One system processes symbols like letters, words, math problems, calendars, maps, etc. They called these visualizations *logogens*. The other system processes people, places, and events in life or a story; these images are called *imagens*. Logogens are organized sequentially, whereas imagens are organized holistically.

In the previous paragraph, I said that memory is typically encoded visually. But there are other ways of processing and remembering information, as is sometimes the case in aphantasia, a term used to describe people who cannot voluntarily make pictures in their minds. However, others struggle with memory and, thus comprehension, their entire lives, never finding a way to compensate for the lack of visualization skills.

Generally speaking, both visualization systems should be equal. However, some people show a significant strength in one and a significant weakness in another. On rare occasions, I have seen some children who appear to have deficiencies in both areas that mask the opposing processing weakness.

Children who struggle to see logogens, or symbols, in their minds are often described as Dyslexic. While children who struggle to see imagens, or pictures and movies, in their minds are often described as Hyperlexic. If visualization problems are the cause of reading struggles or comprehension struggles, respectively, there are other patterns we will see.

Children identified as dyslexic by this one definition will have trouble with reading fluency, spelling, memorizing math facts, and general memorization. They usually process best when information is presented holistically through a "big picture" approach. They also typically enjoy art. But there are other subtypes of dyslexia and the diagnostic code does not distinguish between them.

Meanwhile, children defined as Hyperlexic, in this case, would have trouble with remembering and thus comprehending a story. However, they usually have extreme strengths or interests in letters, words, logos, maps, calendars, and an ear for music. They also learn best when information is presented sequentially.

We will discuss these concepts more in a later chapter, but let's get back to Piaget.

The Formal Operational Stage

At twelve years of age, children typically enter the last stage of Piaget's theory of Cognitive Development: the Formal Operational Stage. This is when abstract reasoning skills begin to develop. This is also the point in development where I become less concerned about differences in processing. Reaching this stage means that enough systems in the brain have been wired up (even if they haven't been wired up in the way we would expect) to support abstract reasoning skills. Simply put, it means that despite any challenges in a child's development, he or she has found a way to wire around that problem. We no longer have to be concerned about additional challenges and accommodations outside the ones we have already experienced.

In Summary

This chapter included a lot of research and the names of several educational psychologists. Although it is nice to understand the development of theories regarding how cognition develops, there are other places we can learn about these ideas.

For example, every single one of these ideas is also represented in Charlotte Mason's final book, *Towards a Philosophy of Education* (written in 1921), including the "Dual Coding" theory, which wasn't developed until 1971.

This makes me wonder if Charlotte Mason had been able to use today's developmental rating scales, might she have conceptualized education differently, especially when students display developmental differences? I believe she would have based educational placement on development, which is why one of the first things I give parents is a developmental rating scale.

I need to know where a child's cognitive development *actually* is, not where we *think* it is based on their age or our biased observations. And the best way I can determine that is to see what they are capable of in various areas such as communication, daily living, social, and motor skills. I, personally, prefer using a developmental rating scale called the Vineland Adaptive Behavior Scales. I have found the patterns of scores in the Vineland manual to be quite valuable, especially in identifying concerns about hearing. I also always test children using the Vineland's motor skills section regardless of age, even though it isn't used to calculate the overall score in children over six years of age. Still, it is the difference among the subscores, and not the overall score, that gives us the most insight as to where that lowest level of development might be. And it is the lowest level that is most important because it shows us where the child is most comfortable working.

Chapter 9

Physiological Needs are More Than Just Skin Deep

"I fear the reader may be inclined to think that I am inviting his attention for the most part to a few physiological matters – the lowest round of the educational ladder. The lowest round it may be, but yet it is the lowest round, the necessary step to all the rest. For it is not too much to say that, in our present state of being, intellectual, moral, even spiritual life and progress depend greatly upon physical conditions. That is to say, not that he who has a fine physique is necessarily a good and clever man; but that the good and clever man requires much animal substance to make up for the expenditure of tissue brought about in the exercise of his virtue and his intellect. For example, is it easier to be amiable, kindly, candid, with or without a headache or an attack of neuralgia?"
- Charlotte Mason

The next thing I often give parents is a Child Development Questionnaire, a 15-page document with extensive questions about a child's developmental history. It is a document I continually update as I refine which questions are the most useful.

Since psychologists receive very little medical training, I

asked local medical professionals to share their intake forms with me. The intake forms I found to be the most helpful came from alternative medicine practitioners. They often do not rely as much on labs and must be more thorough in their questions. I ask about the child's health history as well as the health history of close family members, including what has been tried, what has worked, and what has not. I also ask about the family's cultural and religious values to ensure I honor their values, and that is just the first page!

I also ask more traditional questions on a psychological intake form, such as prenatal and postnatal information and early childhood development, including speech, educational history, and behavior.

But what is particularly unusual is that I also ask questions about a wide variety of bodily systems. I ask quite a few questions about bowel movements and include the Bristol Stool Chart. I also ask questions about the following physical systems: skin, skeletal, endocrine, circulatory, pulmonary, otolaryngology (ENT), odontology (dentistry), immune, and nervous systems. I also evaluate lifestyle and nutrition because what we put into and expose our bodies to dramatically impacts how we feel.

But why do I do this? I am not a medical doctor, and it is not appropriate, nor is it my goal to diagnose or treat medical issues. However, a psychologist must ensure underlying medical conditions are ruled out before considering a psychological diagnosis. Most of the time, we assume that the child's pediatrician has ruled out any underlying medical concerns.

However, I have found that things are often missed, especially for children with developmental differences, that might impact sensory processing and their communication of those symptoms. In fact, it is unusual when I see a child with academic challenges who has no underlying medical concerns!

Medical care creates a number of challenges and barriers

especially for Autistics. Our different sensory processing and communication needs are often not considered. And we are often brushed off as hypochondriacs when expressing our observations of symptoms because we come off as anxious and overly sensitive. Both of those traits are hallmarks of Autism and do not indicate the absence of physiological issues.

Even trauma and emotional disturbances have physiological responses that cause symptoms. Just because we don't understand everything about how the body works doesn't mean physiological issues can't be responsible for the symptoms we notice.

We are designed to grow and learn. It is only when something disrupts the growth and development of the body that growth and learning does not happen.

Albert Einstein once said, "The only thing more dangerous than ignorance is arrogance." Human beings are afraid of the unknown. As a professional, I know just how tempting it is to hide behind research studies and assessments, pretending we are all-knowing. It is natural for us to attempt to fool ourselves into believing everything is knowable with our advanced degrees, research, and assessments. But the reality is that we know very little. Our greatest tool as professionals is the observations of our clients and their parents.

The best doctor I ever saw said to me the first time I met him, "If Mom says something is wrong, we look until we find it." Why "Mom is crazy" is seen as an acceptable conclusion when we are presented with things we do not understand is beyond me. Parents should be seen as equal partners due to their unique insights and observations and the influence they wield over their children. I can accomplish far more by partnering with a parent than by partnering with a teacher because a parent's impact is so significant. This is why I prefer to work with homeschooled families. As Charlotte Mason said, "Mothers work wonders once they are convinced that wonders are demanded of them."

So what am I looking for when I read people's answers to the Child Development Questionnaire? I am looking for any past or present symptoms or events that affect more than one bodily system, no matter how minor. When I see symptoms in two or more systems, it is a good indication that there may be an underlying medical issue. Why two or more systems? In the world of immunology, it is understood that when two or more systems are involved, it ceases to be a localized issue and represents a reaction of the immune system. Some of the more common physiological symptoms I see reported are constipation, diarrhea, bleeding gums, eczema, and copious amounts of earwax, all of which are signs of inflammation in different parts of the body.

It would take an entire set of encyclopedias to thoroughly discuss all the many possibilities for physiological issues. Therefore, I want to spend the rest of this chapter talking about the one thing that comes up most often that we, as parents, have the most control over: Nutrition.

Nutrition

I once taught a class on nutrition to children at a particular religious organization. The class wasn't focused on specific nutrients or diets, as that is outside my area of specialty. Instead, we discussed the idea that what we put into our bodies affects how well our bodies function, and I compared poop to the Biblical analogy of the Fruit of the Spirit. The kids loved me! The parents were a little taken aback though! However, they could not argue with the fact that what we put into our bodies impacts what comes out.

Sometimes, our best indicator of what our bodies need is the symptoms our bodies express, which include far more than just poop. That expression can consist of changes in our skin, behavior, hair, nails, joints, gums, and countless other bodily symptoms. Of course, it would be nice if I could just tell you what the perfect diet is for all children. But that isn't possible. All children are different and have different experiences that impact their biology. What we need can dramatically change over time, either due to changes in age or experiences. And some peoples' systems are generally more sensitive to changes than others. Just as some cars need premium gas or they will leave you stranded on the side of the road, some bodies need a premium diet to keep them running optimally. Also, like cars, we require the right balance to run efficiently.

When I see inflammation across at least two bodily systems, I recommend looking at the child's diet *first*. With the significant increase in allergies and autoimmune conditions in recent years, it makes sense to start there.

For example, based on research by the Mayo Clinic, a positive blood test for celiac disease increased 450% from 1950 to 2000.[1] This is particularly disturbing as the blood test for celiac disease is known to have a high rate of false negatives. And according to research, as much as 95% of children with celiac disease remain undiagnosed.[2]

Stool testing for celiac disease is controversial, with proponents on both sides. However, this is an important avenue of research because it takes, on average, seven years for most people to get a diagnosis of celiac disease. In that time, a significant amount of damage can be done. And in the case of children, who develop so rapidly, this can lead to challenges in development that can never be entirely undone.

No matter which avenue you choose to help you find the cause of inflammation, the elimination diet remains the gold standard. The elimination diet can be as simple as removing one food at a time. But it can also require following a particular diet that removes multiple foods and then slowly adds some foods back to see which ones cause a reaction.

Despite the many types of allergy tests available, there are still so many things we don't know about the immune system. Again, "the only thing more dangerous than ignorance is arrogance."

Anxiety and the Immune System

Another point of interest is that there seems to be a higher instance of autoimmune conditions among Autistics than among the general population. However, I cannot support that claim with scientific research because most studies focus on what causes Autism instead of understanding our health needs.

Research always seems to focus on finding a "cure" for Autism, but the identification of a gene or other "cause" of Autism leads us again down the slippery slope of eugenics. History shows us it is far more likely that we would be eliminated through prenatal testing and abortion like those with Down Syndrome.

I think one of the most promising theories on why Autistics might experience higher rates of autoimmune conditions is the research on Adverse Childhood Experiences (ACEs).

Vincent Felitti, MD, and Robert Anda, MD, created the Adverse Childhood Experiences survey containing just ten different questions on ten different types of adversity. They then had patients complete the survey as part of their research study. The patients were identified as successful individuals with all the advantages that make success more accessible, so they assumed the scores would be relatively low. However, the results were shocking, as detailed in this summary in *Childhood Disrupted: How Your Biography Becomes Your Biology* by Donna Jackson Nakazawa:

> But the number of "yes" answers turned out to be far higher than anyone had predicted. Two-thirds--64 percent--of participants answered yes to one

or more categories, meaning they had experienced at least one of these forms of childhood adversity before turning eighteen. And 87 percent of those who answered yes to one ACE question also had additional Adverse Childhood Experiences. Forty percent had experienced two or more categories of Adverse Childhood Experiences, and 12.5 percent had an ACE Score of 4 or more. Only a third of participants had an ACE Score of zero ... How many categories of Adverse Childhood Experiences patients had encountered could by and large predict how much medical care they would require in adulthood: the higher one's ACE Score, the higher the number of doctor visits they'd had in the past year, and the higher their number of unexplained physical symptoms. People with an ACE score of 4 were twice as likely to be diagnosed with cancer than someone with an ACE Score of 0. For each ACE Score an individual had, the chance of being hospitalized with an autoimmune disease in adulthood rose 20 percent. Someone with an ACE Score of 4 was 460 percent more likely to be facing depression than someone with a score of 0. An ACE score of 6 and higher shortened an individual's lifespan by almost 20 years ... those with ACE Scores of 7 or higher who didn't drink or smoke, and who weren't overweight, diabetic, and didn't have high cholesterol, still had a 360 percent higher risk of heart disease than those with an ACE Score of 0.

Nakazawa says that when we go into red alert, the body dumps essential nutrients such as vitamins, minerals, neurotransmitters, amino acids, hormones, etc., into the bloodstream to help us face the crisis at hand. Once the crisis is over, the body then excretes the remaining essential nutrients that it didn't use out through the urine.

These essential nutrients are the things that make it possible for the immune system to work effectively. But what if this is a chronic situation? What if, as a child, you cannot effectively determine what is safe and what is not?

In this situation, we would experience the same problem as described in the folk song, "There's a Hole in My Bucket" in which Henry repeatedly sings, "There's a hole in my bucket, dear Liza, dear Liza." Only in our case, instead of leaking water, we lose electrolytes, leading to chronic dehydration worsened by drinking more water. This could also explain the anecdotally higher instances of Postural Orthostatic Tachycardia Syndrome (POTS) in the Autistic community, as many people with POTS experience symptom relief through the supplementation of salt tablets.

This has been a heavy topic to consider but the good news is that there are things we can do to prevent our immune systems from deteriorating.

In the next chapter, we will discuss Safety Needs and how we can better support those needs.

Chapter 10
Safety Needs = Self Care

"[Everyone] needs something to love, something to think about, and something to do every day."
- Charlotte Mason

After meeting children's physiological needs, our next most important job is meeting our children's need for general safety and security.

We saw in the previous chapter how trauma can impact our biology. But what qualifies as trauma that is significant enough to affect our physiological health? The answer is anything that causes your body to go into "fight, flight, freeze, or fawn."

Most people are familiar with flight-or-fight, an automatic stress response that occurs when a person perceives a threat, prompting them to either stay and fight or to evacuate the danger zone as quickly as possible.

But a *freeze* response makes a person feel frozen and unable to act against a threat. This can often happen with Autistics because our sensory pathways can be prone to overload. This is why some Autistics lose the ability to speak when stressed.

A *fawn* response is commonly seen in people who have experienced abuse or chronic manipulation and presents as people-pleasing. Manipulation is a tool or weapon, depending on your perspective, chronically wielded at children. Be vigilant against using manipulation, especially with children because most of the time we don't realize that we are doing it. It is natural to want to exert some control over the chaos of our world, but we don't always realize the power we wield over children.

Let's also consider for a moment the potentially traumatic impact of differences in sensory processing. I often like to describe my sensory processing experiences as an Autistic person as being like the scene in the movie *Indiana Jones and the Last Crusade* in which Indiana Jones has to take "a leap of faith" by stepping out over a deep chasm. Until he takes that first step, he cannot see that there is a bridge because it is camouflaged. It is a fantastic moment in the movie, but constantly having to take a leap of faith is a terrible place to live.

To me, that is what it is like to experience differences in sensory processing as an Autistic person. This alone can be traumatic without additional stressors, such as being misunderstood, unable to communicate, learning differences, or lack of acceptance. All of these are challenges faced regularly by Autistic individuals regardless of appearance.

In fact, an Autistic Social Worker who works primarily with Autistic adults reports he has only met one Autistic that didn't exhibit trauma-induced behavior. This is why it is so challenging to diagnose Autism in adults because symptoms of childhood trauma and symptoms of Autism look very similar!

As a rule, a traumatic experience is anything that causes you to experience a trauma response. And this varies significantly from person to person because our perspectives and experiences differ greatly. But if trauma is so personalized, how can we tell when a child has experienced trauma, especially if the child cannot communicate effectively?

Thankfully, there are quite a few things we can look for to

help us determine when a child has experienced trauma. Unfortunately, it won't tell us specifically what the trauma is. It could be some of the physiological needs we discussed in the previous chapter. It could be an underlying medical condition or a lack of having basic needs met, like food, water, clean air, etc. It could be inadequate shelter, clothing, or good sleep. Having all of these basic needs met helps us feel safe and secure. And as we mentioned before, our sensory inputs dictate how we experience the world around us. Thus, they must contribute to our feelings of safety and security.

We all want our children to feel safe and secure, but we should be aware that there is no way to ensure our children feel safe and secure at all times.

And some non-traumatic stress is vital for growth. Without some stress, we do not develop properly. Like a plant raised inside a greenhouse, we will wither from the elements if we have not experienced stressors to help us grow strong. We want children to experience just the right amount of stress that they are developmentally ready for. This kind of stress should not send them into fight, flight, freeze, or fawn. So what are some signs that a child might be experiencing developmentally inappropriate stress?

When I read a family's Child Development Questionnaire, what are some of the things I look for to determine whether or not a child feels safe and secure? I look for trouble sleeping, nail-biting, teeth-grinding, nervous or disruptive behavior, distraction, hyperactivity, any sign of previous trauma or significant life changes, sensory processing differences, constipation, dehydration, and inflammation. One of these signs alone would not be enough to warrant concern that the child might not feel safe and secure. However, the more signs I see, the more I become concerned that the child might be experiencing anxiety.

Our world is highly patterned. We can see mathematical patterns all over the natural world. And if you look carefully enough, you can also see patterns in behavior. That is what I am looking for when I read the answers in a Child Development Questionnaire, the possible patterns that might reveal what needs aren't met. High scores on Internalizing and Externalizing Behavior Scales on the Vineland can also be a sign of stress and anxiety.

If, like most parents, you notice some of these signs in your children, you might be wondering what you can do to support them better. We will talk about several things you can do throughout the rest of this chapter. But the one thing that most Autistic adults wish their parents would have done and the one thing that will make the most difference is the same: Learn to meet your own physical and safety needs (and that includes going to therapy)! We adults do not do this very well, and we teach by example.

In fact, I am setting a bad example right now. I blocked off an entire day to try and make a lot of progress on this book. I did not sleep well the night before. I fed myself coffee and donuts and wondered why I felt a bit jittery by evening. (But it was Pumpkin Spice Coffee and Pumpkin Spice Donuts!) And I have had a severe lack of balance in my day. (And just so you know, I am planning to take the next two days off to soak up all the things I need to bring myself back into balance.) Why do we do this to ourselves? I know I am not the only one.

So often, we feel like whatever the task is, it must be done by a set date, or the world will fall apart. Or we might tell ourselves that we don't deserve a break until we have accomplished x, y, and z, no matter how tired we might be. We often put our kids' needs ahead of our own, and even when we do take time for ourselves, we cannot let go of our worries and concerns. Turns out, though, that when I take better care of myself, my kids are happier and more secure. So if you can't do it for yourself, do it for your kids!

This is a very important point. In fact, it is the point of this entire chapter and will allow us to move into the next chapter regarding Self-Esteem.

When we continually neglect our physiological and safety needs, it says, "I'm not valuable enough." It says, "My value comes from what I do, not who I am." Sometimes supporting ourselves means getting in to see a counselor to unpack unhealthy values we have absorbed. Sometimes it means setting boundaries to protect ourselves, even with our children. It can also mean rediscovering what brings us joy. And sometimes, it means learning how to play again! Play is not an extracurricular activity that you only do if time allows. Play is an essential part of living! It is how we maintain developmental gains in our gross and fine motor skills. But, more than that, play is an opportunity to relax and quit worrying for a little while!

Often when parents, especially mothers, hear the term "self-care," they automatically think it has to be expensive or time-consuming and, therefore, not accessible to them. And, indeed, sometimes expensive or time-consuming things are not accessible when a parent has a high-needs child to care for. And why is that? It is because parents generally love their children and are willing to pour everything they have into making their child's life a little bit easier. However, much like the oft-repeated airplane analogy, you must put on your own oxygen mask before you can help anyone else.

But seriously, if you live this life, you know that even if you want to put your oxygen mask on first, you still have significant limitations. Maybe much of your income goes toward medical bills and/or therapies. Perhaps you are the primary caregiver for a child who cannot be left unattended for safety reasons. But there are still ways to prioritize your own needs. I am not sure who originally coined the phrase "Sabbath Moments," but maybe this phrase will give you a visual of what I am talking about. Below are a few examples of what a "Sabbath Moment" might be for you:

- Dishwashing Mindfulness: Focus on the feel of the water and the dishes as you wash them. See if you don't begin to relax just a bit.
- Enjoy a good audiobook (preferably with noise-canceling headphones) while watching your child. There are some great free audiobooks at librivox.org.
- Do a kids' yoga video with your child. You can find some free yoga videos at Cosmic Kids Yoga on YouTube.
- Learn to play with your child by imitating what they do instead of trying to organize the play into a goal-oriented objective.
- Find a sensory activity that you find satisfying and let yourself spend some time losing yourself in the experience. Whether it is playing with a pop-it, enjoying time in a pool (even a kiddie pool), peeling glue off your fingers, or playing in water beads, try to figure out what you find satisfying!
- Enjoy a leisurely lunch enjoying all of the smells and textures.
- Try to find a friend or relative who can come into your home and give you a break, even if all that means is once a week you spend 30 minutes sitting in a closet eating chocolate and listening to your favorite music!
- Recognize that cell phones are a tool and that sometimes a simple mindless game on your phone can help you decompress while still keeping an eye on your child. No need for mom guilt about not being fully present!

The things we have discussed thus far can also work to varying degrees for children. The key is learning which sensory inputs can help them calm their bodies because each person is different. As much as I would like to spend some time on how we can heal trauma, sometimes this is not possible when we are children. Once again, this is why cognitive development is essential! One of the reasons children are sometimes traumatized by movies, events, or even ideas is due to a lack of complete brain development, which doesn't typically occur until a person's early twenties. With time, they will be capable of processing those traumas.

In the meantime, some of the best things we can do include loving them, protecting them, and providing them with coping strategies and the gift of time.

But suppose that is still not enough to help their bodies calm down. In that situation, I suggest exploring options like Hydroxyzine, which has been well-documented as being a safe, non-dependent medication for treating anxiety in children.[1] I also always suggest looking into different therapeutic approaches to support, like Eye Movement Desensitization and Reprocessing (EMDR), which can help them move memories from the limbic system, or the reactive portion of the brain, into the prefrontal cortex. EMDR can move memories from the part of the brain that causes a chronic fight, flight, freeze, or fawn response and move them to the prefrontal cortex, where further processing can happen as the individual is ready. Given the severe physiological consequences of anxiety, we must address the sense of anxiety and work to increase feelings of safety and security.

But have you noticed that everything I suggested on the list above is free or low-cost? I, too, have been there. Even today, we still can't do some of the things I would like to do because we chose to invest in our kids' health and development when they were young, which cost us dearly. And I would make that same investment choice again every single time because it has been worth the opportunity to watch our kids grow and develop in a more healthy way! Some investments are still worthy, even if they don't make sense financially, especially if it involves your children's future!

Let me tell you a story about someone else who knew the worth of investing in a child's future. Haym Salomon was a Jewish man who immigrated to the American colonies shortly before the start of the Revolutionary War. He became a passionate defender and financier of the Sons of Liberty. He was imprisoned by the British twice and nearly died for his involvement. He loaned more than $650,000 (approximately $16 million in today's money) to the fledgling new government of the United States as it struggled to win the Revolutionary War. In a book called *Haym Salomon: Liberty's Son*, Shirley Milgrim wrote about a scene in which Salomon's wife asked him if he had saved anything as an inheritance for their children. Haym replied,

> Yes, a country where they'll be free to differ in the way they worship God and still enjoy the friendship of other people. I want most to leave the children an opportunity for happiness equal to that of the other citizens of a new nation and a feeling that they are as important a part of the new nation as anyone else.

Salomon died penniless just a few years after the Revolutionary War ended. Generations of Salomon's family have asked the U.S. government for repayment of that initial $650,000 loan, but, to this day, they have not received a single penny. Still, Haym Salomon understood that sometimes an investment might not seem to make sense financially, but if it leaves a legacy for your children, it is worth it.

Life can sometimes be really unfair. And it can feel impossible to live in those moments. During those times, when I feel like I don't have anything left to give, these words from Charlotte Mason have been life-giving to me:

> [Everyone] needs something to love, something to think about, and something to do every day.

I learned that if I looked for something to love, something to think about, and something to do, I could find peace in even the most difficult of circumstances. It is really all about shifting our perspective, which is why practices like mindfulness, praying a rosary, doing martial arts or yoga, and meditating are so essential.

I realize that not every approach is for every person, but find a practice that helps you to listen within. Find a practice that lets you observe your own sensory experiences, let go of the stressors your mind has created, and come home to yourself.

Chapter 11

Self-Esteem = Love and Belonging

"The world needs a sense of worth, and it will achieve it only by its people feeling that they are worthwhile."
- Fred Rogers

People often ask me what they can do to bolster their child's self-esteem. The answer is nothing. Self-esteem comes from within, from the self. However, we can do things to help children have a sense of love and belonging. The home atmosphere goes a long way toward shaping our children's expectations of self-worth as well as how others should treat them.

So how do we create a healthy atmosphere of love and belonging?

First, let's begin by looking at an ancient blessing that has been part of Western culture for thousands of years and what it might offer us. The Biblical Priestly Blessing found in Numbers 6:24-26 is a blessing from God to bestow a sense of love and belonging on the Israelites.

May God bless you and keep you.

> *Let God shine His face upon you and grant you grace.*
> *Let God lift His face towards you and grant you peace.*

Many Jewish parents say this blessing over their children every Friday night (the Jewish Sabbath), and Christians often sing it to each other in their Churches. It even appears in pop culture as the Vulcan greeting "Live long and prosper" from Star Trek.

Rabbi David Fohrman suggests that we can view the three lines of this blessing as three building blocks to providing our own children with a sense of love and belonging.

The first line focuses on blessing and keeping. The word *blessing* is associated with the idea of increasing. As women, we carry our babies in our wombs with the idea of increasing that baby so that it can be born to a life independent of our body. On the other hand, the word *keeping* implies the opposite kind of energy. Whereas *blessing* is a positive energy in nurturing the child's growth, *keeping*, or safeguarding, is a negative energy in keeping that child protected and safe from harm. Both words, *bless* and *keep*, come from the same Hebrew root, the word for womb.

Interestingly enough, the word for compassion also comes from the name of this most motherly organ in the human body. And having compassion is nothing more than feeling such a strong sympathy with another being that we desire to nurture and safeguard that person. This *blessing* and *keeping* is something we, as a society, begin doing when children are first being formed and we continue to *bless* and *keep* them until they are one day able to do those things for themselves. We are ensuring their physical, emotional, intellectual, and moral well-being so that one day, as adults, they will be able to safeguard themselves from both external and internal dangers.

The second and third lines of the Priestly Blessing mention the face: *"shine His face upon you"* and *"lift His face towards you.*

The first time we hold our child, we smile and shine our face lovingly down upon that child. The child hasn't done anything yet, but we love them simply because they are ours. That is the definition of grace, a love freely given. It is a top-down kind of love that depends only on one person, the parent. There is no plan to "fix" the child because they are not "good enough." This kind of unconditional love leads to a child's growth because it imbues the child with the confidence to look his mother in the face, to babble, to take those first steps, to walk away from his mother, to meet other people, to try new skills and new activities. It is the one thing each child needs more than anything else.

In the third line of the Priestly Blessing, our gaze shifts from looking down upon our children to looking them in the face. As our children grow, they begin to take on more and more independence, making more decisions for themselves. We begin to meet their gaze instead of looking down at them, and as they make choices, some of which we will not always agree with, we try to give them a sense of peace or love without guilt or judgment. This kind of love is much more difficult for a parent to give, to let go and accept your children even when they disappoint you. As we begin this "letting go" of our children, we begin to focus less and less on nurturing and protecting *them* and, instead, begin to focus on nurturing and protecting the sacred space of our relationship. This ensures that the relationship is always available for both of us.

You might think, "This all sounds lovely, but how do we bring these ideas forward to modern times?" We will tackle that question using Rabbi Fohrman's method of the three building blocks mentioned above.

In the first line of the Priestly Blessing, there is a lot of vocabulary that, in today's world, might sound very traditional or even patriarchal. However, regardless of the type of parental identity or views you might have, the fact remains that children experience the consequences of prenatal and perinatal trauma well into adulthood. This period is a fragile time for development. And I do not believe that we, as a society, take enough time to consider the potential impact of trauma on growth and development even though plenty of research exists to support those findings. Even something as simple as a mother's stress level during pregnancy correlates with doubling a child's risk of emotional or behavioral issues.

Does this mean we should blame the mother for any problems that may arise? Absolutely not! There are so many things beyond our control that happen during prenatal and perinatal development. However, it is crucial to recognize that there are things that do fall within our control and that we are responsible for the atmosphere we actively create, not only for a baby to be born into but also to be nurtured as that baby grows. That also means we have it within our power and, what's more, it is our responsibility to create an atmosphere where healing can begin.

But where and how do we begin this work? With ourselves. Autistic adults often say they wish that, when they were growing up, their parents would have seen a therapist. We all have baggage and trauma; it comes with living life. But we are much better people and parents when we work to deal with our own baggage and trauma so that we are not parenting from a place of reactivity.

Now, as we move on to the second line of the Priestly Blessing, you might be thinking, "This whole 'shining your face lovingly down on your child without any plans to fix them' sounds great, but how do these ideas help me get my child to do all the things they need to do in a day?"

To answer this question, we will once again turn to British educator Charlotte Mason. In her third and fourth principles of education, Mason said:

> The principles of authority on the one hand and of obedience on the other, are natural, necessary, and fundamental; but—These principles are limited by the respect due to the personality of children, which must not be encroached upon whether by the direct use of fear or love, suggestion or influence, or by undue play upon any one natural desire.

What this means is that we all live under some kind of authority. For example, you can't just go out and kill people without consequences. And the same goes for other infractions like stealing because authority must consider the needs of others.

But Mason also points out that when we are in a position of authority, we cannot act the part of a tyrant and manipulate others into doing what we want them to do. And she reminds us that parents are naturally placed in a position of authority over their children and, therefore, should not manipulate them.

Manipulation can take many forms and can even be unintentional and well-meaning. But that doesn't make it okay. Mason lists the more common methods used for manipulating children, including love, fear, suggestion, influence, and natural desires. We must respect each person's individuality, no matter how small they may be.

To explain the importance of respecting individuality, we will use one of the ethical principles in yoga: *asteya*, or non-stealing. When we consider whether or not we steal, many of us will quickly answer 'no'. But consider: do we ever steal someone's opportunity to learn or communicate their thoughts? It has been my experience that we, as individuals, and as a collective society, steal from our own children in a thousand subtle ways each day.

This realization that we sometimes steal from our own children brings us to the real question: do we trust God, the universe, or even our children to walk the path of learning and life laid out for them? Or are we afraid of how we will feel depending on where that path takes our children? I think this is very often the case, and it is why parents often work so hard to try and "fix" their children. They fear the hurt they might feel when seeing their children walk a path different from what they perceive as desirable. This fear is quite common among parents because of their attachment to their children, and we will come back to address this fear more fully when we get to the third building block of the blessing.

But staying with the second building block for now, of shining our faces down lovingly on our children, what will we use to motivate our children if we can't use fear, love, suggestion, influence, or natural desires? We find the answer in the first building block, the atmosphere we create, with yet another quote from Charlotte Mason: her fifth principle.

> Therefore, we are limited to three educational instruments—the atmosphere of environment, the discipline of habit, and the presentation of living ideas. [Our] Motto is: "Education is an atmosphere, a discipline, and a life.

Mason describes education as "an atmosphere, a discipline, and a life" because we learn from people, things, events, habits, and "life" in general. In other words, we learn from the atmosphere in which we live!

We want to be mindful of the atmosphere we live in, but we also don't want to try and create a perfect and artificial environment. First, it will not produce what we want. Like the greenhouse plants not suited to live outside in the elements, a perfectly curated environment with no stressors will not prepare our children for life outside our home. Second, children will see through our attempts to create a perfect and artificial environment and still suffer the effects of the baggage we have tried to sweep under the rug. We can only provide our children with a healthy atmosphere by living authentically.

But what do I mean by living authentically? It means knowing our principles and living by them, and yes, sometimes that can mean going to therapy! To know our principles cannot mean aligning ourselves with an outside list of expectations. Principles are the core feelings that mean the very most to you that remain unchanged even when no one else is around.

Let me give you an example of what I mean. These are some of my own principles. You will have to discover your own for yourself, but perhaps these will get you thinking about what some of your principles might be.

Amy's Principles

- Behavior: We are respectful, kind, and appreciative to all creatures, including ourselves.
- Activity: We habitually prioritize what we believe is most important, not perfection.
- Parenting: Children are born persons worthy of respect and personal freedom.
- Spirituality: We take time daily to connect with our own spirits and spiritual practices.
- Education: We regularly partake in a rich and varied feast of ideas.
- Health: We listen to our bodies daily and provide them with what they need.

As you can see, these values don't contradict any specific approach a person might take because they do not tell you what to do. Rather, they inform the spirit with which you make choices.

Rules, on the other hand, both spoken and unspoken (such as in the form of social skills), are more particular and arbitrary. And they tend to work best in only specific settings and cultures. And indeed, rules are essential for an orderly society because they tell us how a particular social group will choose to interpret principles into action. It is why people in different areas of the world, social classes, races, religions, and neurotypes interpret the same behaviors differently! But rules can also be challenging to follow if they are not explicitly stated, and even uncomfortable if they require you to refrain from being authentic. For short periods, you can 'mask' or be inauthentic, but as mentioned at the end of Part 1, everyone needs a home where their soul can be at peace with themselves.

Children especially feel the weight of rules because children often have very little say in what the specifics of those rules are going to be. And sometimes, children cannot participate in that decision-making process due to their current level of development. But it makes it all the more incumbent on us, as adults, to be mindful of the rules we choose to enforce, whether directly or indirectly.

Research shows that the ideal number of rules is three because that is approximately how many rules children can remember and the number that adults can consistently enforce. With such a small number of rules, we must be mindful of the ones we choose to help our homes run smoothly. One trick we can use to minimize the number of rules needed is to word them in such a way that it tells the child what *to do* instead of what *not to do*.

When our children were younger, our three household rules were very concrete and focused on basic safety skills such as:

- We stay out of the fireplace

- We sit on our bottoms in chairs
- We go outside with an adult

You might be able to guess where we got the inspiration for such rules: our children and their antics! As they got older, our three household rules became more abstract and focused on the things that we deemed necessary for our home to run well:

- We are kind
- We are truthful
- We do our work

These kinds of rules require a lot more teaching because they can vary greatly from one circumstance to another.

But what happens when a child breaks one of these rules? Better yet, what happens when an adult breaks one of these rules? In our home, someone else, whether a parent or child, will privately bring it to the person's attention. It is then incumbent upon that person to make amends. And generally speaking, that is about all that happens.

When parents treat their children with kindness, they often get kindness back from their children. When we as parents make sure that the children in our home treat each other with kindness, they are more inclined to develop the habit of being kind to each other.

Now, it is true that sometimes a person is not in a state to receive this constructive criticism or make amends. In those cases, we find it important to help that person return to a state where they can receive constructive criticism well and are willing to make amends. Within the Autistic community, this is referred to as a meltdown..

Anyone can have a meltdown. A meltdown is when you reach such a point of imbalance that you experience an overload of your senses. It can happen when you are hungry or tired, but it can also occur when you have heard your child repeat the same exact phrase for the hundredth time. Ideally, we recognize this imbalance before it leads to a meltdown, but sometimes we don't. Sometimes this is because things are hitting us too fast for us to process, like when you receive multiple pieces of bad news one after the other. Other times we end up melting down because we forget to take time to listen to our bodies.

When we inevitably reach a meltdown, we have passed the point of being able to utilize coping strategies or do anything other than react. It is at this point that the family mobilizes to provide needed support. Sometimes this means helping a child utilize coping strategies when unable to do so themselves. Sometimes this looks like encouraging a parent or child to take a break in a place of sanctuary from the overload. Other times this looks like one parent making sure the children feel well supported while the other parent is processing through their meltdown.

How we talk about these moments after they occur is important because they teach our children how to become supportive spouses and parents. As an Autistic adult, I still occasionally have meltdowns, but not as often as I used to. One particular meltdown has become known as "Hurricane Amy." I was so incredibly overloaded that I actually upended furniture to meet my need for heavy-work sensory input. However, our children had seen me support them through meltdowns so often that this time they could assist their dad in helping me, which was an amazing thing to see. My daughter texted me, saying, "I know you are upset, and I am happy to help you. But you are being too loud for me right now. When you are quieter, I will help you." When I ran out of energy, they all came into the room, hugged me through my tears of frustration, joked about Hurricane Amy's destruction, and helped me pick up the room. Afterward, my daughter made us each a cup of tea, and we sat down to discuss why I was overloaded. Later, once I had de-escalated entirely and returned to a more balanced state, I apologized and worked to make amends for any discomfort I might have caused. Home is where people love you just the way you are, support you through hard times without taking it personally, and set the standard for what kind of treatment you will tolerate from others.

When we began this chapter, we started by talking about the three building blocks for creating homes where people feel loved and a sense of belonging.

The third and final building block of the Priestly Blessing is learning to look our children in the eye as they grow into themselves and to give them a sense of peace or love without guilt. We are so attached to our children that we are very often afraid to let go, but we must set them free because otherwise, they cannot grow into the gift that they are: themselves!

But how do we get over this fear? We learn to overcome this fear by working on it when our children are still relatively young, by learning to look for ways to say "Yes" instead of "No" as often as we can.

Our family therapist once told me when our children were younger how impressed she was with how free and yet secure my children felt. She likened it to sending a child out into a great forest to play; all the while, the child never realized there was a fence enclosing the "forest" to keep him safe. That "forest" was the testing ground where my children learned who they were, challenged their skills, and learned to conquer their challenges. And the "fence" is what allowed me to say "Yes" instead of "No" as often as I could.

But to have a fence, we have to think ahead. We cannot be parenting from a reactionary place. And this is the work you have to do. You must know your principles, choose your rules and habits carefully, and build fences to protect your child's autonomy.

Chapter 12

Cognitive and Aesthetic Needs = Seeing the Beauty that is All Around Us

"It is as necessary for man to live in beauty rather than ugliness as it is necessary for him to have food for an aching belly or rest for a weary body."

- Abraham Maslow

We are nearing the end of this book and I'm finally going to talk about education! And there is a reason for that. Cognitive Needs, or what we traditionally think of as education, is where most people want to start.

Parents are very often surprised when I start talking about physiological or psychological health issues. But the reality is that almost every time I speak with parents whose children struggle academically, there are almost always some underlying health issues. Although we all constantly go up and down Maslow's Hierarchy of Needs like a ladder throughout our lives (or even throughout the same day!), we must address the most basic needs before addressing higher-level needs.

We cannot educate well enough to bypass basic human needs. We can also cause trauma by ignoring basic needs and skipping ahead to the "truly important work" of education. And I don't just mean the trauma of unmet basic human needs. I also mean the trauma of exposure to ideas before the brain is ready to handle them. This determination of where our children are developmentally is what can prove so challenging to parents and is what we will discuss for the rest of this chapter.

First, we need to start by asking the question, "How do we learn?" It is well-established in neuropsychology that we learn through our senses. Dr. Maria Montessori claimed in the late 1800s that these sensory learning experiences begin at birth, but today we know that these sensory learning experiences start even earlier.

Newborns automatically recognize the smell and taste of their mother's breast milk due to its similarities to the mother's amniotic fluid in utero. Movement in utero serves to help the developing child organize their sensory-motor pathways. Starting at 27 weeks gestation, they are able to hear and remember songs that are played frequently. Throughout our lives, we take in information about the world around us through our senses which our brain then works to process and organize.

These abilities allow us to adapt to our environment. On that point, Maria Montessori was correct and was ahead of her time, for our sensory experiences allow our brains to develop as they should. When one sense cannot function, it leads to significant differences in brain development.

The brain is an incredibly flexible organ that, given enough time, can find ways to rewire around most issues, but it cannot create connections as they were originally intended before a disruption occurred.

When an adult loses their hearing, they must use the motor cortex to learn sign language. However, when a child who is born deaf communicates through sign language, the language center of his brain will light up. We see fewer neural processing differences in adults who lose their hearing because most brain development has already occurred before the brain must rewire in order to learn sign language.

Over time we have worked to improve our ability to support rewiring through the work of Dr. Jean Ayers and Dr. Edgar Rey Sanabria.

Dr. Jean Ayers was an Occupational Therapist who spearheaded the development of what is now known as Sensory Integration Theory. Dr. Edgar Rey Sanabria was the head of the Neonatology Department at Instituto Materno Infantil in Columbia, the first hospital to implement what is now known as Kangaroo Care in NICUs worldwide. Children worldwide owe both individuals a debt of gratitude for how these changes in how we treat children have led to significant improvement in sensory processing development and, thus, learning.

In typical situations, most sensory integration in childhood happens through play. In atypical developmental situations, play can also have a powerful impact on sensory integration, even if extra assistance is required in the form of an Occupational Therapist, Physical Therapist, Speech Therapist, Orofacial Myofunctional Therapist, Massage Therapist, etc.

As Fred Rogers, the host of the children's television program *Mister Rogers Neighborhood*, said,

> Play is often talked about as if it were a relief from serious learning. But for children, play is serious learning. Play is really the work of childhood.

More than a hundred years before Mister Rogers, Charlotte Mason said in her first book, *Home Education*,

> In this time of extraordinary pressure, educational and social, perhaps a mother's first duty to her children is to secure for them a quiet growing time,

a full six years of passive, receptive life, the waking part of it spent, for the most part, out in the fresh air.

More recently, a study published in 2022 in *The Journal of Developmental Psychology* by Durkin, Lipsey, Farran, & Wiesen looked at data from 2,990 children from low-income families who applied to pre-K program sites across Tennessee. The children admitted to the pre-K program sites had lower state achievement test scores in third through sixth grades and more disciplinary infractions, absences, and receipt of special education services.

At a time when the pressure to obtain a good education begins as early as preschool, I believe we may do our children and ourselves a favor by taking to heart Ms. Mason's advice of a "quiet growing time" in those early years.

But what of Maslow's Cognitive Needs? Merriam-Webster defines *cognitive* as "relating to mental activities such as thinking, reasoning, remembering, imagining, learning words, and using language," or, put another way, processing ideas, most frequently presented through some sort of language.

Charlotte Mason speaks to this in her final book, *Towards a Philosophy of Education*:

> For the mind is capable of dealing with only one kind of food; it lives, grows and is nourished upon ideas only; mere information is to it as a meal of sawdust to the body; there are no organs for the assimilation of the one more than of the other.

Therefore, if the mind must feed on ideas, and ideas are presented primarily in language form, we should wait to formally meet a child's cognitive needs until a child has developed pre-reading skills and has thus become fluent in oral language skills.

Charlotte Mason developed a checklist to determine if fluency in oral language skills had been achieved. However, this was no ordinary checklist. It was called "A Formidable List of Attainments for a Child of Six," and accurately assesses pre-reading skills and language development even though it may not seem like that when first viewed (the checklist appears at the end of this chapter for your convenience).

Today, a speech therapist or an assessment of overall development like the Vineland Adaptive Behavior Scales could also help determine oral language fluency skills.

But what do we do if those language skills never develop? We work to find ways to continue building connections with our child and providing a loving, supportive, and enriching environment that encourages growth and learning to happen comfortably.

We can presume competence without pressuring and exposing children to things they may not be ready for by sharing different kinds of art, music, videos, audiobooks, experiences, and activities with them. After all, this is how learning continues to happen throughout our lives, even once formal education has ceased. The key, though, is to consider these activities (that you likely already do) as part of their mental diet and work to ensure a nutrient-rich but well-balanced feast for their developing minds. And, similar to meal-planning, it is essential to consider a child's individual needs and abilities so you don't try to serve a steak to an infant that hasn't developed the teeth and muscles necessary to digest that steak safely.

Skill Subjects vs Ideas

Our next question is, "How do we support our child's cognitive needs once oral language fluency develops, no matter when it happens?"

Traditionally, education begins through instruction in the three R's: reading, writing, and arithmetic. Achievement in reading, writing, and arithmetic does serve a fundamental purpose in the education process, even though they are not how we meet cognitive needs. They provide us with more options to communicate and share ideas with others. And if you think about it, foreign languages, music, art, and even physical activities, also meet this need.

Reading well allows us to read other people's ideas; writing well lets us express and expound upon our ideas. And, of course, being fluent in a foreign language allows us to participate in the exchange of ideas in a different language.

While perhaps less obvious, arithmetic is another vehicle to communicate and share ideas. Arithmetic is the "alphabet" of the "language" of mathematics. Through this alphabet, we describe and theorize about the physical world around us with others, even when they do not speak the same language as us.

Art and music represent more abstract ways of expressing and sharing ideas. Even physical activities like dance, martial arts, yoga, and any handicraft allow for the expression of ideas and communication within our bodies and the world around us.

These are all "skill subjects" that we work to develop, hopefully in a balanced way, to allow for the greatest expansion of our options for communication in this world. But they are not just "skill subjects." They are also opportunities to meet students' aesthetic needs and refine their ability to appreciate the beauty hidden within these subjects.

Some of our world's finest works of art exist as words on a page in the form of poetry. But mathematics also has its own beauty, not just in its orderliness but also in the beautiful things in nature it describes, such as the Fibonacci Sequence.

And it is through a student's efforts to develop fluency in any of the arts that he comes to see and appreciate how beautiful each truly is. David Hicks wrote in his book *Norms and Nobility*:

> The paideutic man's attitude toward such activities as painting, drawing, violin playing, dancing, and acting is amateurish, not professional. He knows that one cannot learn the culture defined by these activities passively. Since culture is the unique property of the participant, not of the spectator, the classical academy resists the modern tendency to select only the most talented for participating. The modern school, to the contrary, frequently regards culture as entertainment, and the educator's cultural mission is taken up with exposing his students to an assortment of entertainments. He hopes to arouse their uncritical appreciation of art without attempting to sharpen their habits of discrimination or to develop their participatory skills.

As Hicks puts it, it is our participation and work to develop our skills in these subjects that help us see the beauty that is all around us. Our purpose is not to outperform others on a test or merely be able to decode. Our purpose is to be able to not only appreciate the beauty but also be able to use those subject areas as avenues for sharing ideas.

So why do we begin students' education with the monotonous nuts and bolts of the three R's without also exposing them to how someone has taken those nuts and bolts to turn them into something beautiful? Why are the arts always the first to go when school boards cut funding? In a world where stress and cortisol levels are through the roof, we cannot afford to cut aesthetics from our classrooms when these are the very subjects that increase levels of oxytocin in the brain, which serves to decrease cortisol levels.

With so much of modern education focused on increasing fluency and raising test scores, are there opportunities available in the curriculum to meet students' cognitive needs, and if so, how? Literature, history, science, physics, etc., all provide opportunities within the curriculum to meet students' cognitive needs. However, the curriculum chosen for lower grade levels often gives minimal attention to these subjects, if they include them at all. Not that other subject areas cannot stimulate cognitive faculties, but with so much emphasis on skill subjects for fluency, there is often not much room left for ideas. When this happens, many students, especially those who struggle with accessibility, end up not getting their cognitive needs met sufficiently.

If we want to meet the cognitive needs of children, we have to start by ensuring that we meet all other basic needs first. Once we have met those basic needs, we also have to include opportunities to foster their curiosity and facilitate opportunities to build relationships with things that spark their interest.

I have had the chance to observe many teachers up close in many different types of schools. Some of them are punching a clock until retirement. Others are frustrated and overwhelmed because they do not have the tools to do the job the school system is asking them to do.

But some teachers truly make a difference and inspire the students they teach, despite the constraints they must work within. How do these talented teachers manage to do this? Why do students fondly remember these teachers even decades later? The secret is quite simple. They take an interest in their students, get to know them, and treat them respectfully. That is teaching and parenting in a nutshell. It is all about relationships. When children have healthy and respectful relationships with important adults, it makes all the difference and can help them overcome great odds.

You might think, "Gosh, that sounds as idyllic as a meadow full of rainbows and unicorns! But how does that work in the real world where things often aren't ideal?"

First of all, this is the most significant disadvantage of public education. Yes, public education provides the opportunity for some children to receive an education they would otherwise not be able to receive. But, it also means that we are very often trying to meet the cognitive needs of children when, in reality, they have foundational physical and emotional needs going unmet that we cannot do anything about. This educational environment can also negatively affect those same children, particularly if other challenges already exist, such as learning disabilities.

As it turns out, learning disabilities are actually a bit of a source of frustration for me because we do not have clear language to define most learning disabilities. And getting a diagnosis doesn't necessarily help the child. The word Dyslexia means "problem in reading." Dysgraphia means "problem in writing." Dyscalculia means "problem with calculation." Dyspraxia means "problem with movement." Those definitions only tell us what we already know: there is a problem!

But to help students, we must ask, "Why are they having trouble? Is there an imbalance in their development that needs support so they can grow and develop more easily? Is there a processing issue blocking them? If there is more than one processing issue blocking them, which should we address first?" We have used these designations for decades because Psychology has, since its infancy, used symptoms to try and find a way to help people. But, as we learn more about how the brain processes information, we will eventually have to change our diagnostic system because many different processing deficits can lead to "a problem in reading" or "a problem in writing."

Of all the various processing issues that come across my desk, the most common imbalance I see is between logogens and imogens, often dubbed Dyslexia and Hyperlexia, respectively (as previously mentioned in the Dual Coding Theory).

By our current diagnostic system, those very different challenges would likely both fall under the category of Specific Learning Disability in Reading. But just that one classification has a plethora of possible processing issues! And because I feel that it is essential to address processing issues in the same order in which they are used in the brain, I will briefly give you an example of the many different steps I go through when determining which areas might cause challenges for a particular student.

The first thing I will investigate is if a student has a language delay. And if they have a language delay, they may not be developmentally ready to learn to read.

Next, I find out if they have had their vision checked. Then, I will ask about how their brain processes what their eyes are seeing. Do the letters appear to wiggle, or does reading make their eyes tired? Then I will ask if they can see words in their minds, and if so, what those words look like. I will also ask what they see in their mind while listening to a story. These questions give me insight into how their brain processes information according to the Dual Coding Theory.

Only after all those steps will I consider an Orton-Gillingham Reading Program. What good is it to try to remediate difficulties in reading if a child does not have the language development necessary to read, cannot see well enough to read, or can't remember well enough to master such a complex skill?

The real question is, "Do any learning disabilities block a child from getting their cognitive needs met until it is fully remediated?" And the answer is only one: language comprehension deficits.

In all other instances, we can use tools to accommodate any

Cognitive and Aesthetic Needs = Seeing the Beauty that is ...

disadvantage. We can read books aloud to children, use audiobooks, or pens that read to you as you scan the page. We can watch videos, use closed captioning, and read graphic novels. We can use pens that record audio when you scribble, speech-to-text, predictive text, spell check, and grammar check. We have so many excellent tools available today to give children access to ideas.

We only need three things to meet the cognitive needs of children: language fluency, invested adults willing to serve as tour guides along the learning journey, and play, lots of play!

"A Formidable List of Attainments for a Child of Six" by Charlotte Mason

1. To recite, beautifully, 6 easy poems and hymns
2. to recite, perfectly and beautifully, a parable and a psalm
3. to add and subtract numbers up to 10, with dominoes or counters
4. to read--what and how much, will depend on what we are told of the child
5. to copy in print-hand from a book
6. to know the points of the compass with relation to their own home, where the sun rises and sets, and the way the wind blows
7. to describe the boundaries of their own home
8. to describe any lake, river, pond, island, etc. within easy reach
9. to tell quite accurately (however shortly) 3 stories from Bible history, 3 from early English, and 3 from early Roman history (my note here, we may want to substitute early American for early English!)
10. to be able to describe 3 walks and 3 views

11. to mount in a scrapbook a dozen common wildflowers, with leaves (one every week); to name these, describe them in their own words, and say where they found them.
12. to do the same with the leaves and flowers of 6 forest trees
13. to know 6 birds by song, color, and shape
14. to send in certain Kindergarten or other handiwork, as directed
15. to tell three stories about their own "pets"--rabbit, dog, or cat.
16. to name 20 common objects in French, and say a dozen little sentences
17. to sing one hymn, one French song, and one English song
18. to keep a caterpillar and tell the life story of a butterfly from his own observations.

Chapter 13

Self-Actualization and Transcendence

"The privilege of a lifetime is being who you are."
- Joseph Campbell

We have finally reached the pinnacle of Maslow's Hierarchy of Needs: Self-Actualization and Transcendence.

It isn't until we reach this top tier that we have everything we need to experience moments of Self-Actualization and Transcendence. Generally speaking, this doesn't happen until at least the teen years or, more likely, adulthood because our brains are still in a significant stage of development until then. And some people never reach the ultimate pinnacle of Transcendence. These are those moments in life when everything seems to line up just right, and you have clarity regarding who you are and what you need to be doing in a larger context. These moments don't often happen because we constantly move up and down Maslow's Hierarchy of Needs trying to address unmet needs.

However, it's not just these rare moments of transcendent clarity that are significant. Self-Actualization, or being in a healthy balance, is also important. Having balance in the different areas discussed throughout this book allows us to reach out to others in a healthy way. Without Self-Actualization, we are just grasping at things that we think might fulfill our more basic needs. Not reaching Self-Actualization is what leads to many unhappy marriages and lives. When for example, we do not feel safe and secure, we feel attracted to others who make us feel safe and secure, even if it is an unhealthy type of security, such as in a cult, gang, or abusive relationship.

Until we reach Self-Actualization for the first time, we have spent our entire lives working to meet our basic needs, but these basic needs all serve as the foundation for social development. We like to think that social development is relatively simple and that we can teach children how to socialize appropriately. But this is genuinely too simplistic. Childhood is about meeting those basic needs to help us know ourselves and prepare us to reach out to others.

To have truly healthy interactions and relationships with others, we must first have:

- our basic physical needs met so that we can focus on things beyond food, water, and shelter
- the security to reach out to others
- the experience of love and belonging to be able to connect and communicate
- the self-esteem to know our own worth and to value the worth and individuality of others
- the cognitive skills to understand others

We need all of these things to allow us to develop well socially.

Professionals often tell us that the way to help our children develop socially is to send them to school, and there is nothing wrong with sending children to school. But, one of the most frequent questions I hear as a homeschooler is, "What about socialization?"

I would like to argue that school is not where we learn the social skills we will use in adulthood. When was the last time you were in a classroom setting full of people all the same age? It was probably high school, if not earlier.

But when did you last go to the grocery store, the post office, or the park, talk to someone older than you, or play with a child younger than you? You have probably done all of those things relatively frequently throughout your life. Those situations are where we learn the social skills we will use throughout the rest of our lives, and those are situations that my children find themselves in frequently as homeschoolers. But, if a school environment is *not* necessary for learning social skills, the question remains, "What kinds of environments are necessary?"

Despite what adults in our lives might have told us as children, when you get to adulthood, you get to choose the people you surround yourself with. Childhood is a time to figure out what kinds of people you would like to reach out to, and the sky's the limit! When deciding who to reach out to, you must ask yourself, "What continent? What country? What region? What culture? What social class? What religion?" etc.

Different groups have distinctly different social skills, and not everyone will feel at home with the same groups. Just because your parents raised you in a particular culture, religion, or social class does not mean you must stay there. You aren't your parents; what is right for them may not be right for you.

One of the most challenging things about being a parent is learning that your children may not enjoy the same things you do. It may be difficult to support and guide them through choices you would have never chosen. To do this well, we need to focus on our own self-actualization as much as possible, or we will be parenting from a place of reactivity without the ability to respect our child's individuality. (As an aside, I firmly believe everyone needs a family therapist to help them avoid parenting from a place of reactivity without the objectivity that a therapist can offer!)

So how do we teach our children social skills if we are unsure what kind of social environment we are preparing them for? The short answer is that we don't teach our children social skills. Beyond meeting more basic needs in Maslow's Hierarchy of Needs, we can only partner with our child socially.

But what do I mean by *partner*? So often in our society, children are regarded as second-class citizens with the expectation that when we say "Jump!" it is their job to say, "How high?" That is not partnering. That is compliance training. And teaching children compliance is the greatest enemy of self-advocacy. It can lead our children to become victims of abuse if they are in the habit of always complying with the wishes of adults and others in authority. Partnering, on the other hand, looks like walking through social situations *with* your child, and you can do this in many different ways.

One of the things I used to say to myself over and over again when my children were younger was, "Mind your own mat, Amy." The reason I said this is because it would remind me of the two rules I have in my Family Yoga classes.

The first rule is for the children, and that rule is to "Be kind to the people and things in the room" (and yes, we often have to have conversations about what that means). The second rule is for the parents, and that rule is to "Mind your own mat." This means I expect parents to give their children the freedom to connect and relate to yoga in whatever way works for them, so long as they are being kind to the people and things in the room.

Those rules have informed my parenting also by teaching me that while I must ensure that my children are held accountable for being kind toward others, I must not steal their opportunity to learn how to interact socially with others.

But how do you ensure that your children are being considerate of others while also minding your own mat?

Sometimes you do have to physically stop your child from running into someone and potentially knocking them over, and sometimes you must address something your child said in the moment because it was hurtful. But, often you can take the opportunities before social events to talk with your child about what they might expect to see, how people might talk or act, what others might be expecting, etc., without placing any pressure on them for how they should behave.

And when you are leaving a social outing, you can talk with your child about whether or not they enjoyed themselves and what they noticed. If they mention something didn't go very well, you can use that opportunity to explain to your child how other people might have interpreted your child's behavior. Children are often not aware of how other people interpret their behavior and sometimes need to be told. You can also suggest different ways your child could try responding in similar future settings to achieve a different result. In other words, become your child's cultural translator!

Making a point of introducing your child to a variety of settings will give you even more opportunities for these kinds of conversations. You might even ask your child if they noticed differences in how people behave in different settings and discuss why that might be.

I remember having a similar discussion with my children years ago when I decided I wanted them to experience the symphony. I had grown up occasionally having the opportunity to go to symphonies, plays, and operas. Though my parents had started their marriage in the working class, they had risen throughout my childhood to the upper-middle class. And even though I had four brothers and sisters, my parents chose to send my siblings and me to a small private school where I made friends with other students whose families had season tickets to the Orpheum Theater. I also worked in a jewelry store in high school that sold to some of the upper echelons of society in our city, so I had the opportunity to have experiences that my parents did not have growing up. But as an adult, I have made choices congruent with a solidly middle-class lifestyle, even though I didn't realize it at the time. I thought I was just falling in love and getting an education in the areas that appealed to me, but I was also choosing the social class to live in that felt the most comfortable.

But getting back to going to the symphony with my children, I explained to them what behaviors they should expect to see while they were there. It evolved into a fascinating discussion about how our jobs, schedules, leisure activities, etc., all vary greatly depending on our social class and how they will have to decide which social class is most comfortable for them to live in. I still love the opportunities that an upper-middle-class lifestyle afforded me. And, through our state's homeschool scholarship, I have occasionally introduced my children to opportunities that we might not have been able to otherwise afford. But even if I sometimes enjoy those types of upper-middle-class activities, I still prefer to live a middle-class lifestyle because that is where I feel most at home.

These conversations with your children are significantly more helpful to *you* than your child because they will offer insight into what kinds of social settings are comfortable for your child and which types of social skills might be most valuable for them to develop. But they can also help your child feel more secure in their ability to choose the social situations that appeal to them without feeling inadequate. Of course, the more personal and firmly held your preferences are for certain social situations, the harder this will be. That is why I strongly recommend that everyone have a good family therapist to help them sort through these feelings. And, of course, there are other times when there will be more than one person in a family with almost completely opposing preferences, in which case you will have to work hard to compromise and offer some amount of personal freedom.

Strongly held feelings make it difficult to allow wiggle room for your children's preferences. I know of no social situation more fraught with this than religion. And this is particularly challenging for American families.

Joseph Campbell wrote that cultural traditions, such as coming-of-age traditions, are the glue that holds a society together in a changing world. The United States is a nation of immigrants from many different cultures, and in many ways, we do not have the same cultural traditions that other countries do. A large percentage of immigrants came to the United States in search of religious freedom and believed it would be "a land where troubles melt like lemon drops ... and the dreams that you dare to dream really do come true," (a line from "Over the Rainbow," a song written by children of Jewish immigrants).

Many of the coming-of-age traditions that do exist in American society come from our various religious backgrounds: Confirmation, Quinceañera, Bar Mitzvah, Bat Mitzvah, Rumspringa, etc. Without cultural coming-of-age traditions, we are inclined to cling even more fiercely to our religious traditions for stability in an ever-changing world.

The best advice I can offer in these types of challenging situations is to remember the principles you have established for yourself and your family. Take the time to evaluate what is *really* most important to you, how to preserve what is most important to you, and how to let the rest go. Hopefully, your children and your spouse are at the top of your "most important" list, since they are people you have made a sacred commitment to. Take the time to have open conversations with your family, where everyone can express their feelings and preferences without judgment. Children can't always provide insight into what explicitly bothers them or what they prefer. However, allowing them to see that you are listening sets a powerful example of how to positively relate to others.

Look for ways to compromise. Perhaps you have a child who needs a small and quiet worship setting, and you could find a small house of worship. Or maybe you avoid telling stories from your religious tradition until your child is older and their brain is more prepared to handle stories with content we might not typically consider to be child-friendly. For example, I found the story of the Ten Plagues to be quite terrifying as a child. My thinking was, "Wait! Does God still kill the firstborn? I am the firstborn! I am not so sure I am comfortable with this!"

Whatever you choose regarding religion as a social situation, you want your child to see the beauty of your tradition and that it is a place where they feel loved and accepted for who they are. And if you don't have a chosen religious tradition, look for traditions that you can emphasize to connect your child to their larger community, culture, and values.

Even with the best of intentions, we can accidentally trigger trauma symptoms in our children if they are exposed to things that terrify them into a fight, flight, freeze, or fawn reaction. Abuse of any kind causes fragmentation within ourselves. The deeper and more personal the abuse, the more fragmentation. What we call our souls is entwined in the very nature of who we are, which is why we must be careful to guard our children's souls.

These fears of our children are worth paying attention to and taking seriously. It is a child's way of communicating to us that they have an unmet need, and in this case, it is likely a safety need. One of the best steps you can take is to find other adults who can relate to and comprehend your child's experience. An Autistic adult can often give insights into why an Autistic child might be reacting the way they are to a particular situation. Those adults have the advantage of having a fully developed brain and can thus express their feelings more easily than our children can at their stage of development.

Community with others *like ourselves* is vital. It protects children from feeling like something must be wrong with them because they are so different from everyone they see around them. And it provides parents with needed support in understanding their child's perspective! We all have strengths and weaknesses that can influence our parenting, but there are others in our communities that have different strengths and weaknesses. Having those people in our lives is the antidote that can help bring balance to keep us from passing on our generational traumas. We might be able to manage meeting the lower needs in Maslow's Hierarchy of Needs alone in a cave. But Self-Actualization and Transcendence require community and embracing the ties that bind us together.

Chapter 14

Putting It All Together: Case Studies

"It is good to have an end to journey toward, but it is the journey that matters in the end."
- Ernest Hemingway

We have finally come to the end of our journey together through this book. We started this journey from many different places and perspectives, but together we have traversed a myriad of different ideas, which I hope have given you some thoughts to chew on. Yes, many of those ideas have been more philosophical, but change begins with ideas.

But how do you apply these ideas beyond just the broad brushstrokes? On my website, we have educational Boost Packets that dig deeper into specific topics and offer practical help, and I am working on publishing more educational resources for both parents and professionals!

But I also want to spend the rest of this chapter providing some examples of specific situations to show how we might apply these ideas in those situations. Even though each of the following case studies is entirely fictional, they are examples of common patterns that I see in many students.

Case Study: Jon

Jon is a five-year-old boy diagnosed with Autism. His parents are completely overwhelmed by his impulsive and destructive behaviors. Their doctor has suggested ABA, but they are uncertain about the therapy. Given his behavioral issues, Jon's parents are looking for advice about teaching Jon in a homeschool setting.

Jon's parents list various symptoms on his Child Development Questionnaire, including bleeding gums, 'chicken' skin, fluctuating stool consistency, anal itching, and bedwetting. Although bedwetting is considered normal for Jon's age, the presence of symptoms in more than three bodily systems could indicate an immune problem. When asked if Jon has any known allergies or has ever had any health concerns, Jon's parents answered, "No, but we did try removing some foods from his diet because someone told us that helps kids with Autism. However, Jon became very defensive and even hostile, so we stopped."

Due to Jon's traumatic response to having foods removed, I recommend they get a referral to an Immunologist for further testing. I also suggest that, rather than removing foods, they begin keeping a food diary. I further suggested they consider creating a 'snack box' of Jon's healthy comfort foods and make it available at all times to give him more control and security regarding his foods. I explain to Jon's parents that many Autistic individuals experience anxiety and trauma due to differences in sensory processing, including food choices, and how that trauma can impact their experience of the world and people around them. I further explain that this anxiety in childhood can cause Autistic children and adults to experience immune issues due to the physiological impact of chronic anxiety.

In the meantime, since Jon is so young, I recommend taking a break from formal schooling while addressing these potential health challenges and taking more of an unschooling, child-led, and play-based approach to education for a little while.

Case Study: Sarah

Sarah is an eight-year-old girl. Her parents are very concerned because she is still not reading and wonders if she might be Dyslexic. They have no other concerns, but they mention offhand that she also struggles with memorizing math facts. Looking at her Child Development Questionnaire and her Vineland Adaptive Behavior Scale, her development appears to be pretty typical, with no apparent language delays. Her achievement scores, though, tell a very different story. Her reading and writing scores are all low, as well as most of her math scores. However, her listening comprehension scores and math problem-solving skills are quite good! She shows classic signs of a Specific Learning Disability in Reading, often referred to as Dyslexia.

Her parents recently took her to an ophthalmologist to ensure she could see correctly. When asked, Sarah reports that the letters do not wiggle when she reads, and her eyes do not get tired. She does say that sometimes her brain gets tired when reading, though! When asked if she can visualize letters in her mind and, if so, what color or texture they are, Sarah looks at me quizzically, confused about what I asked. I recommend that Sarah's parents halt instruction in reading. Instead, I suggest they use my *Building Reading and Spelling Skills* manual to address weaknesses in Rapid Automatized Naming.

I also recommend that, for the rest of the year, they focus on reading aloud to her about various subjects, including math, to capitalize on her exceptional listening comprehension skills!

When I see Sarah again a year later to reassess, Sarah is not only reading, but she is now reading at grade level! Her numerical computation scores are still a little low, so I recommend that Sarah's parents apply the *Building Reading and Spelling Skills* manual to Sarah's math difficulties, which will help her visualize math problems. I also recommend they consider switching from Saxon Math to Math-U-See because Math-U-See generally seems to help students who can see the big picture but struggle to visualize symbols.

Case Study: William

William is a 16-year-old boy. He loves reading and excels in most subjects in school, but he prefers to avoid driving and is struggling significantly in math, which brought his parents to me.

When asked about his early education, William's parents report that he taught himself to read at three years old. They also say handwriting is a struggle, and William adds that he prefers to type. However, William's mother is quick to point out that William does not type the correct way and that his early-developed habits in typing seem to have stuck.

I ask William and his parents if they had ever heard of Hyperlexia or Nonverbal Learning Disability, and they reply that they have never heard of it. I explain that while these are not official diagnoses in the current Diagnostic and Statistical Manual, they describe the pattern in William's learning strengths and weaknesses.

Nonverbal Learning Disability simply represents more of a weakness in visual-spatial skills than in verbal skills. Deficiencies in visual-spatial skills can impact one's ability to move through space fluidly, drive comfortably, write, and understand mathematical concepts. While these skills are not impossible for William, we do need to be mindful of ways we can support the development of skills that are important to him and how we can make accommodations for skills that are not as important to him.

Knowing that William is interested in attending college, I recommend that we focus our efforts on strengthening his math abilities and suggest William use a math curriculum called Life of Fred. William's greatest weakness in math is not fluency or computation, but mathematical reasoning skills, and Life of Fred specifically focuses on building mathematical reasoning skills using William's greatest strength: reading.

I also recommend that William play more video games to improve the specific spatial skills that are also used in driving but to also consider applying to college campuses with good public transportation options to decrease the necessity of driving while dealing with so many new changes and stressors.

Case Study: Anne

Anne is a nine-year-old girl who was born prematurely at thirty weeks gestation which resulted in medically-induced trauma and differences in sensory processing. This has created high levels of anxiety, leading to symptoms of Pathological Demand Avoidance (now called Protective Demand Avoidance, renamed by Dr. Mona Delahook).

Then, at six years old, the COVID pandemic hit, and Anne experienced many changes to her routine very quickly and developed social anxiety and more fears relating to her health.

Anne's parents are extremely concerned about her inability to return to school and participate in recreational activities with friends. They mention that besides the significant levels of anxiety Anne is experiencing, she is also having fainting spells. Upon further questioning, her parents do not think these fainting spells correlate to periods of increased anxiety. Looking at her Child Development Questionnaire, I notice that constipation is a chronic issue. And even though Anne's eating habits are good, her parents are concerned that Anne doesn't eat or drink enough and that she craves too much salt in her food. At this point, I ask her parents if they had talked to her doctor about some of these symptoms, and they reply that they assumed it is all connected to the anxiety.

I affirm that these kinds of symptoms often occur with anxiety, but still recommend consulting with her doctor in case the severe levels of anxiety have potentially developed into Postural Orthostatic Tachycardia Syndrome. I also recommend they talk to their doctor about whether medication might be an option for supporting her through this time of intense anxiety so that she can better use her coping strategies. And because I suspect that nausea might be a symptom of Anne's anxiety, I suggest that her parents ask her doctor about the possibility of using a combination of Zofran and Hydroxyzine to reduce anxiety and help her eat and drink more.

Beyond that, I provide her parents with resources for a variety of coping strategies, such as counseling to help her process her feelings and develop more coping strategies, yoga and mindfulness to help her calm her mind, and massage therapy to help work out the tension she is holding in her body.

I also recommend taking a break from formal education for a little while, as it is challenging to learn when you are constantly on high alert. Instead, I recommend her parents take more of an unschooling and child-led approach to education for the rest of the year. I remind them that with their support, she can easily catch up and re-enter the school system with her friends or choose to continue homeschooling on her timeline.

Our priority should always be supporting her physical and mental health.

Case Study: Nick

Nick is Autistic and identifies as a transgender male. Nick was born female with the given name of Nicole.

Nick's mom suffered from severe postpartum depression, so Nick's paternal grandmother, the only relative who lived near them at the time, took over the caregiver role for much of Nick's first five years of life. Unfortunately, when Nick was five, his grandmother suffered a heart attack and died suddenly. Nick is now twelve years old and has significant attachment and post-traumatic stress from these experiences. Nick's father has been a stable influence, but he is often gone for work. Nick's parents are also concerned that they may have missed some needed support.

Nick's family wants to support Nick as well as they can, and they have already provided Nick with access to a therapist to help Nick explore and process his feelings. Nick's therapist seems to be doing excellent work acknowledging Nick but also allowing Nick to truly explore any underlying feelings. The counselor suggested that they begin their work by leaving all labels at the door and working through Nick's feelings first, and then if Nick wants to pick a label back up, that's fine. But the goal is for Nick to explore all feelings and have help communicating those feelings.

While looking at the Child Development Questionnaire, Nick's parents indicate that Nick has celiac disease and describe Nick as being rather wiry and flexible. I am not surprised to see this pattern of symptoms. Many Autistics can be wiry and flexible due to Ehler-Danlos Syndrome (EDS), which is often a comorbidity of Autism. So that is one possible explanation;

however, it is also not uncommon for Autistic teens to try to control physical change in their bodies by maintaining a low body mass index (BMI). However, given the celiac diagnosis, I believe EDS may be a concern because celiacs have an estimated 50% greater incidence of having EDS,[1] so I recommend Nick's parents get a referral from their doctor to see a specialist.

Having EDS could further complicate things for Nick's lifelong medical care. EDS could put Nick at greater risk of bruising more easily, having a far more difficult time healing and closing wounds, and a greater chance of organ prolapse or even tearing. It also impacts physiological development, including bone development, because bones depend on proper muscle stress to grow correctly. Care for EDS typically includes managing symptoms, preventing further complications, and avoiding surgery whenever possible due to potential risks. Nick's celiac disease could also negatively impact overall development because the body may not absorb adequate nutrition early in life due to the damage celiac disease can cause to the digestive tract. Thankfully, Nick is only twelve years old, and with proper diagnosis and care, Nick's parents have the opportunity to provide the best chance for long-term health!

I recommend Nick continue seeing the therapist to work through and process feelings. I also recommend that their family doctor have Nick evaluated for EDS. If EDS is suspected, Nick should begin receiving ongoing care based on the advice of the medical team, which could include ongoing chiropractic care, massage therapy, and working with a physical therapist and/or personal trainer who is familiar with EDS and can help develop the muscles needed to hold joints together in a healthy way.

Case Study: Emma

Emma is a ten-year-old girl without any diagnoses, but her parents are concerned that she just doesn't seem to be making progress with her schoolwork. I have her parents fill out my Child Development Questionnaire and the Vineland Adaptive Behavior Scales. We also include additional testing with the Wide Range Achievement Test and the Listening Comprehension subtest from the Wechsler Individual Achievement Test.

Emma's health seems very good, and I see no developmental concerns from either the Child Development Questionnaire or the Vineland Adaptive Behavior Scales. As for the achievement tests, Emma's subtest score for word reading is precisely where I would expect it to be, but her reading comprehension, spelling, and math computation scores are below average. Her listening comprehension subtest places her at two years below her age level.

Given that academic delays seem to be the primary issue, I return to the Child Development Questionnaire for more details. Emma's parents report that she seems to have a natural ear for music and she also enjoys drawing. They assume that anything artistic is her thing!

Emma also reports that when reading or listening to a book, she sees pictures in her mind, but they do not move and are not always in color. When spelling a word, Emma has to attempt to sound it out, even familiar words that she reads and writes a lot, because she can only see a few letters in her mind at a time.

I tell Emma's parents I cannot be 100% certain based on the information collected, but I believe she has two opposing processing weaknesses that compensate for each other to the point it masks both problems. I suspect that Emma is both "dyslexic" and "hyperlexic." Her parents feel this perfectly explains their daughter; however, they also look confused, as if they are thinking, "How can Emma be both dyslexic and hyperlexic?"

I explain to Emma's parents that in this context, I am using the term dyslexic for a person with weak symbol imagery and the term Hyperlexia for a person with weak concept imagery.

I have noticed a pattern in children who appear to have both weaknesses. The children often present with a smattering of strengths and weaknesses that are characteristic of both processing extremes. For example, dyslexic children are usually gifted artistically and have exceptional comprehension. In contrast, hyperlexic children are often exceptionally gifted in music and seem to have a natural ability for spelling and memorizing facts. Emma, on the other hand, is gifted artistically and musically but struggles with spelling and comprehension.

I recommend that her parents continue with their Charlotte Mason approach to education but focus on including more picture books, graphic novels, and movies to provide visual support while we work to strengthen her processing weaknesses. And because they are homeschool parents on a single income, I recommend they start with my *Building Narration Skills Manual*. Once Emma reaches a maintenance level, they can then add my *Building Reading and Spelling Skills Manual*.

Case Study: Jack

Jack is a 7-year-old boy diagnosed with Autism due to a known gene mutation. Jack does not speak much, and when he does speak, it appears to mostly include echolalia, or repeating phrases. He is currently in speech therapy and occupational therapy. His parents are confused and frustrated about how they should proceed in homeschooling Jack when he does not seem to behave and learn like other children.

I have Jack's parents fill out my Child Development Questionnaire and the Vineland. Aside from some mild symptoms related to his gene mutation, Jack appears to be in excellent health. He also does not appear overly anxious, though he does appear to be in Piaget's Sensorimotor Phase of development with strong preferences for certain types of sensory inputs and activities such as playing with squishy items and heavy work inputs like jumping. Jack's scores on the Vineland indicate that most of his developmental skills are falling in the birth to 2 years range, the same range as Piaget's Sensorimotor Phase of development. Other than that, Jack appears to be a happy and well-loved child!

When I meet with Jack's parents, I tell them that they have done a fantastic job of supporting Jack so far, as evidenced by his happy demeanor and positive relationship with his parents. I also point out how pleased I am to see that his physical development is progressing in such a healthy way. However, I also acknowledge that, as parents, they also want to continue to deepen their ability to connect with Jack as much as possible.

I ask Jack's parents if they have ever heard of Gestalt Language Processing. They reply that they have not. I then explain that it is a relatively new area of study within the field of speech pathology. Researchers noticed that some children, instead of beginning by learning a few words, will instead begin speaking with whole phrases. They will then use these phrases in different contexts, and even if the phrase may not fit the context perfectly, it can still express the feeling the child wants to convey.

Jack's mother lights up at this point and says that she has seen Jack do this, but she didn't realize other children did this too! I then suggest that his parents connect with a speech therapist who specializes in Gestalt Language Processing. I suggest that speech therapy, combined with videos, books, and shared attention, would fit Jack's current language development needs perfectly.

I also encourage his parents to avoid working on forming

letters in occupational therapy and instead focus on developing fine and gross motor skills and meeting sensory needs. I also suggest they consult with an occupational therapist who specializes in primitive reflexes.

For any remaining academic requirements for their state, I suggest using passive activities such as playing a video in the background like *Wild Kratts* for science or *Super Why* for language arts. I am also careful to point out that even though we will not be pushing Jack academically, that does not mean they should not presume competence, and they should, by all means, include Jack in all life activities that interest him, just as they have been doing his whole life!

But primarily, I tell his parents that they are doing an excellent job of honoring Jack's personhood and hopefully, with some assistance from professionals in these newer areas of expertise, they will be able to enjoy even deeper connections with Jack! And finally, I encourage them to join my Special Needs Membership group so they can access ongoing support as he continues to grow and change!

Love and Balance

Hopefully, these case studies have given you some insight into how you can make the ideas presented in this book work for you! There are Jons, Sarahs, Williams, Annes, Nicks, Emmas, and Jacks all around us just waiting for us to hear what their bodies are trying to communicate.

I truly believe that all children deserve the respect we so freely give to adults and that we should all be willing to acknowledge and accommodate for the individual needs of others. It is what we should do as part of the human family: love and support each other. When we see the possibilities in others, we can truly love them just as they are.

Thank you for taking the time to really hear what I have

tried to communicate in this book. If I could leave you with only two words to sum up the heart and soul of this book, they would be *love* and *balance*.

> "Next to love, balance is the most important thing."
>
> — John Wooden, Basketball Coach

If we lead with love and balance, we can't go wrong.

Join the BOOK DISCUSSION!

SPECIAL NEEDS KIDS are people too!

SEEING THE POSSIBILITIES THROUGH A NEURODIVERSE LENS

Join a live book discussion with

Amy Bodkin, EdS

Autistic Adult & Special Needs Consultant

Scan the QR code for more info!

About the Author

Amy Bodkin is a Consultant and Public Speaker serving families with needs that fall outside the norm. She is uniquely qualified to help families with a wide variety of special needs. Amy is an Autistic Adult, has an Educational Specialist degree in Educational Psychology with an emphasis in Neuropsychology, a Master's degree in Educational Psychology, and she homeschools her two Autistic kiddos.

In all of her work, Amy takes a developmental approach paired with the educational philosophy of Charlotte Mason that "children are born persons" and are worthy of the respect due to all persons. You can check out all that Amy does to advocate for the better treatment of children at her website, AmyBodkin.com. It's as easy as ABC: Ally, Boost, and Connect! Ally with Amy through her podcast, "Special Needs Kids Are People Too!" Get a boost with her educational resources. And connect through her Special Needs Membership group as well as private consultations for families and professionals.

Amy lives in Florida with her husband, two children, two cats, and a dog. You can also find her on Facebook and Instagram.

Other Resources by Amy Bodkin

Special Needs Membership
Special Needs Consultation for Families
Special Needs Consultation for Professionals
Planning, Organizing, and Documenting Your Homeschool
Workshop: Supporting Special Needs Families in Your Co-op
Special Needs Development Guide

See all of our resources at:
AmyBodkin.com

Charlotte Mason's 20 Principles

1. Children are born persons.
2. They are not born either good or bad, but with possibilities for good or evil.
3. The principles of authority on the one hand and of obedience on the other, are natural, necessary, and fundamental; but—
4. These principles are limited by the respect due to the personality of children, which must not be encroached upon whether by the direct use of fear or love, suggestion or influence, or by undue play upon any one natural desire.
5. Therefore, we are limited to three educational instruments—the atmosphere of environment, the discipline of habit, and the presentation of living ideas. The P.N.E.U. Motto is: "Education is an atmosphere, a discipline, and a life."
6. When we say that "education is an atmosphere," we do not mean that a child should be isolated in what may be called a 'child-environment' especially adapted and prepared, but that we should take into account the

educational value of his natural home atmosphere, both as regards persons and things, and should let him live freely among his proper conditions. It stultifies a child to bring down his world to the child's level.

7. By "education is a discipline," we mean the discipline of habits, formed definitely and thoughtfully, whether habits of mind or body. Physiologists tell us of the adaptation of brain structures to habitual lines of thought, i.e., to our habits.

8. In saying that "education is a life," the need of intellectual and moral as well as of physical sustenance is implied. The mind feeds on ideas, and therefore children should have a generous curriculum.

9. We hold that the child's mind is no mere sac to hold ideas; but is rather, if the figure may be allowed, a spiritual organism, with an appetite for all knowledge. This is its proper diet, with which it is prepared to deal; and which it can digest and assimilate as the body does foodstuffs.

10. Such a doctrine as e.g. the Herbartian, that the mind is a receptacle, lays the stress of education (the preparation of knowledge in enticing morsels duly ordered) upon the teacher. children taught on this principle are in danger of receiving much teaching with little knowledge; and the teacher's axiom is, "what a child learns matters less than how he learns it."

11. But we, believing that the normal child has powers of mind which fit him to deal with all knowledge proper to him, give him a full and generous curriculum; taking care only that all knowledge offered him is vital, that is, that facts are not presented without their

informing ideas. Out of this conception comes our principle that,—

12. "Education is the Science of Relations"; that is, that a child has natural relations with a vast number of things and thoughts: so we train him upon physical exercises, nature lore, handicrafts, science and art, and upon many living books, for we know that our business is not to teach him all about anything, but to help him make valid as many as may be of— "Those first-born affinities that fit our new existence to existing things.
13. In devising syllabus for a normal child, of whatever social class, three points must be considered: (a) He requires much knowledge, for the mind needs sufficient food as much as does the body; (b) The knowledge should be various, for sameness in mental diet does not create appetite (i.e., curiosity); (c) Knowledge should be communicated in well-chosen language, because his attention responds naturally to what is conveyed in literary form.
14. As knowledge is not assimilated until it is reproduced, children should 'tell back' after a single reading or hearing: or should write on some part of what they have read.
15. A single reading is insisted on, because children have naturally great power of attention; but this force is dissipated by the re-reading of passages, and also, by questioning, summarizing and the like. Nor is the accuracy of this statement limited to clever children or to children of the educated classes: thousands of children in Elementary Schools respond freely to this method, which is based on the behavior of mind.
16. There are two guides to moral and intellectual self-management to offer to children, which we may call

'the way of the will' and 'the way of the reason.'

17. The way of the will: Children should be taught, (a) to distinguish between 'I want' and 'I will.' (b) That the way to will effectively is to turn our thoughts from that which we desire but do not will. (c) That the best way to turn our thoughts is to think of or do some quite different thing, entertaining or interesting. (d) That after a little rest in this way, the will returns to its work with new vigor. (This adjunct of the will is familiar to us as diversion, whose office it is to ease us for a time from will effort, that we may 'will' again with added power. The use of suggestion as an aid to the will is to be deprecated, as tending to stultify and stereotype character. It would seem that spontaneity is a condition of development, and that human nature needs the discipline of failure as well as success.)

18. The way of reason: We teach children too, not to 'lean (too confidently) to their own understanding'; because the function of reason is to give logical demonstration (a) of mathematical truth, (b) of an initial idea, accepted by the will. In the former case, reason is, practically, an infallible guide, but in the latter, it is not always a safe one; for, whether that idea be right or wrong, reason will confirm it by irrefragable proofs.

19. Therefore, children should be taught, as they become mature enough to understand such teaching, that the chief responsibility which rest on them as persons is the acceptance or rejection of ideas. To help them in this choice we give them principles of conduct, and a wide range of the knowledge fitted to them. These principles should save children from some of the loose thinking and heedless action which cause most of us to live at a lower level than we need.

20. We allow no separation to grow up between the intellectual and 'spiritual' life of children, but teach them that the Divine Spirit has constant access to their spirits, and is their Continual Helper in all the interests, duties and joys of life.

Works Cited

Chapter 1

1 Guan, J., & Li, G. (2017). Injury Mortality in Individuals With Autism. *American Journal of Public Health*, *107*(5), 791–793.
2 Kirby, A. V., Bakian, A. V., Zhang, Y., Bilder, D. A., Keeshin, B. R., & Coon, H. (2019). A 20-year study of suicide death in a statewide autism population. *Autism Research*, *12*(4), 658–666.
3 Villarreal, V. R., Katusic, M. Z., Myers, S. M., Weaver, A. L., Nocton, J. J., & Voigt, R. G. (2024). Risk of Autoimmune Disease in Research-Identified Cases of Autism Spectrum Disorder: A Longitudinal, Population-Based Birth Cohort Study. *Journal of Developmental & Behavioral Pediatrics*, *45*(1), e46.

Chapter 2

1 Rider University. (2021, September 15). *Are IQ Tests flawed? Rider Professor Explores the Dark History of IQ Tests for TED Platform*. Rider University.
2 Harris, J. E. (2020, October 14). *Why Buck v. Bell Still Matters*. Bill of Health; Petrie-Flom Center, Harvard Law School.

Chapter 3

1 Cook, M. (2022, February 15). *Iceland Lashed over Down Syndrome Record at UN*. BioEdge.

Chapter 4

1 Ravilochan, T., Ravilochan, V., & Kessler, C. (2021, August 18). *Could the Blackfoot Wisdom That Inspired Maslow Guide Us Now?* Medium.
2 McDermid, C. D. (1960). How Money Motivates Men. *Business Horizons*, *3*(4), 93–100.
3 Bridgman, T., Cummings, S., & Ballard, J. (2019). Who Built Maslow's Pyramid? A History of the Creation of Management Studies' Most Famous Symbol and Its Implications for Management Education. *Academy of Management Learning & Education*, *18*(1), 81–98.

4 University of California, Davis. (2020, July 24). *The Wood Wide Web: Underground Fungi-Plant Communication Network*. The Aggie Transcript.
5 McLeod, S. (2024b, January 24). *Maslow's Hierarchy of Needs*. Simply Psychology.

Chapter 5

1 Bruns, P. F. (2015). *Dear Prudence: The Story Behind the Song*.

Chapter 6

1 Yellowhorn, E., & Lowinger, K. (2017). *Turtle Island: The Story of North America's First People*. Annick Press.
2 Library of Congress. (n.d.). *Under Attack: Immigration and Relocation in U.S. History*. Library of Congress.
3 Valenti-Hein, D., & Schwartz, L. D. (1995). Sexual Abuse Interview for Those With Developmental Disabilities | Office of Justice Programs. *National Criminal Justice Reference Service, 153917*. U.S. Department of Justice National Criminal Justice Reference Service (NCJRS) Virtual Library.

Chapter 9

1 Mayo Clinic. (2009, July 2). *Celiac Disease Four Times More Common Than In 1950s*. ScienceDaily.
2 Sahin, Y. (2021). Celiac disease in children: A review of the literature. *World Journal of Clinical Pediatrics, 10*(4), 53–71. National Center for Biotechnology Information.

Chapter 10

1 Pardini, C. (2003, September 29). *Hydroxyzine for Anxiety: How It Works, Side Effects, & Dosages*. Good Rx Health.

Bibliography

Abraham Joshua Heschel, & Heschel, S. (2011). *Essential writings*. Orbis Books.
Al-Musawi, M. J. (2007). *The Arabian nights*. Barnes & Noble Classics.
Alcott, L. M. (2014). *The complete Little Women series*. e-artnow.
Austen, J., & Kinsley, J. (1998). *Sense and Sensibility*. Oxford University Press.
Ayres, A. J. (2005). *Sensory integration and the child: understanding hidden sensory challenges*. Western Psychological Services.
Ballantyne, S. (2013). *The paleo approach: Reverse autoimmune disease and heal your body*. Simon & Schuster.
Baraka, A. (1963). *Blues people: Negro music in white America*. Perennial.
Beethoven, L. van, & Hannes, A. (2006). *Music Masters: The Story of Beethoven in Words and Music* [Audio CD]. Music Masters.
Bharati, J. (2011). *Living the yoga sutras: Practical translations and discussions*. Abhyasa Ashram.
Bowman, K. (2017). *Move your DNA: Restore Your Health Through Natural Movement* (2nd ed.). Propriometrics Press.
Bulfinch, T. (2014). *Bulfinch's mythology: The age of fable, the age of chivalry, and legends of Charlemagne*. Canterbury Classics.
Campbell, J. (1968). *The hero with a thousand faces*. Pantheon Books.
Campbell, J., & Moyers, B. D. (2012). *The power of myth*. Turtleback Books.
Campbell-Mcbride, N. (2012). *Gut and Psychology Syndrome*. Medinform Publishing.
Cloud, H., & Sims Townsend, J. (2004). *Boundaries*. Zondervan.
Cohn, J. (2023). *The Christmas Menorahs*. Lechambon Press.
Cook O'Toole, J., & Holliday Willey, L. (2012). *Asperkids: An insider's guide to loving, understanding and teaching children with Asperger syndrome*. Jessica Kingsley Publishers.
Cook, D. (2001). *Taekwondo*. Ymaa Publications.
Crook, W. G., & Crook, C. P. (2006). *The yeast connection handbook*. Professional Books.
Dawson, P., & Guare, R. (2009). *Smart but scattered: The revolutionary executive skills approach to helping kids reach their potential*. Guilford Press.
Delahooke, M. (2019). *Beyond behaviors: using brain science and compassion to understand and solve children's behavioral challenges*. Pesi Publishers.
Dersa, S. (2023). *Homeschooling Wildflowers*. A Homemade Education Press.
Diekman, A. (2023). *Low-Demand Parenting*. Jessica Kingsley Publishers.
Dotterer, C. L., & Alyssa, M. (2018). *Handwriting brain-body disconnect: Adaptive*

Bibliography

teaching techniques to unlock a child's Dysgraphia for the classroom and at home. Author Academy Elite.

Elder, J., & Thomas, M. (2007). *Autistic Planet*. Jessica Kingsley Publishers.

Eliot, L. (2010). *What's going on in there?: How the brain and mind develop in the first five years of life*. Bantam.

Fallon, S., & Enig, M. G. (2005). *Nourishing traditions* (2nd ed.). Newtrends Publishing.

Finkelstein, N. H. (1992). *The Other 1492*. Beech Tree Paperback Book.

Frankl, V. E. (1946). *Man's search for meaning*. Beacon Press.

Frankl, V. E. (2021). *Yes to life: In spite of everything*. Beacon.

Gates, R., & Kenison, K. (2002). *Meditations from the mat: Daily reflections on the path of yoga*. Anchor Books.

Glass, K., & Hicks, D. V. (2015). *Consider this: Charlotte Mason and the classical tradition*. Createspace.

Gogh, V. van. (2022). *Beyond Van Gogh: The Immersive Experience*. Beyond van Gogh. https://beyondvangogh.com

Greene, R. W. (2014). *The explosive child: a new approach for understanding and parenting easily frustrated, chronically inflexible children*. Harper.

Hamilton, E. (2011). *Mythology: Timeless tales of gods and heroes*. Grand Central Publishing.

Hawke, E. (2015). *Rules for a knight: the last letter of Sir Thomas Lemuel Hawke*. Knopf.

Healthed. (2015). *Professor Tony Attwood - Autism in Females*. Healthed. https://vimeo.com/122940958

Hegel, G. (2019). *Georg Wilhelm Friedrich Hegel: The phenomenology of spirit*.

Hicks, D. V. (1999). *Norms & nobility: a treatise on education*. University Press of America.

Hirsh-Pasek, K., & Golinkoff, R. M. (2014). *How babies talk: The magic and mystery of language in the first three years of life*. Plume.

Horn, D. (2022). *People love dead Jews: Reports from a haunted present*. W. W. Norton & Company.

Iḷaṅkōvaṭikaḷ, & Adigal, I. (1965). *Shilappadikaram*. New Directions Publishing.

Jackson Nakazawa, D. (2015). *Childhood disrupted: how your biography becomes your biology, and how you can heal*. Atria Books.

Jensen, A. (2005). *When babies read: a practical guide to help young children with hyperlexia, Asperger syndrome and high-functioning autism*. Jessica Kingsley Publishers.

Jovin, D., Atwal, P., Schofield, J., & Koby, M. (2020). *Disjointed: Navigating the diagnosis and management of hypermobile Ehlers-Danlos syndrome and hypermobility spectrum disorders*. Hidden Stripes Publications, Inc.

Kaplan, A. (2011). *Jewish Meditation*. Schocken.

Katz, P. (2021). *The Art of War*. Canterbury Classics.

Kennedy, J. F. (2016). *Profiles in courage*. Harper Perennial.
Kolk, B. van der. (2014). *The body keeps the score: Brain, mind, and body in the healing of trauma*. Penguin Books.
Kushner, H. S. (2001). *When bad things happen to good people*. Schocken Books.
LaMothe, K. (2006). *Nietzsche's Dancers*. Springer.
Leibovitz, L. (2020). *Stan Lee*. Yale University Press.
Levison, C. (2000). *A Charlotte Mason education: A home schooling how-to manual*. Sourcebooks.
Levison, C. (2001). *More Charlotte Mason education: A home schooling how-to manual*. Sourcebooks.
Little, J. (1973). *From Anna*. Harper Collins.
Livingstone Smith, D. (2012). *Less than human: Why we demean, enslave, and exterminate others*. St. Martin's Griffin.
Lynch, B. (2020). *Dirty genes: A breakthrough program to treat the root cause of illness and optimize your health*. HarperOne.
Marshall, J. (2005). *Quiet Thunder: The Wisdom of Crazy Horse*. Sounds True.
Maslow, A. H. (1999). *Towards a Psychology of Being* (3rd ed.). John Wiley and Sons.
Mason, C., & Lebowitz, R. (2019). *A Philosophy of Education: Annotated Edition*. A Charlotte Mason Plenary.
Meigs, C. (1990). *Invincible Louisa*. Scholastic Book Services.
Montessori, M. (2014). *The Montessori method*. Transaction Publishers.
O'Neal Johnston, A. (2022). *A place to belong: Celebrating diversity and kinship in the home and beyond*. TarcherPerigee.
Riley, R. (2016). *Post-traumatic church syndrome: one woman's desperate, funny, and healing journey to explore 30 religions by her 30th birthday*. Howard Books.
Rogers, F., & Junod, T. (2019). *A beautiful day in the neighborhood: Neighborly words of wisdom from Mister Rogers*. Penguin Books.
Ruttenberg, D. (2022). *On repentance and repair*. Beacon Press.
Sacks, J. (2007). *The dignity of difference: how to avoid the clash of civilizations*. Continuum.
Sadoski, M., & Paivio, A. (2013). *Imagery and text: A dual coding theory of reading and writing*. Routledge.
Sapolsky, R. (2004). *Why zebras don't get ulcers* (3rd ed.). Holt.
Sattar, A. (2018). *Ramayana*. Restless Books.
Schaeffer Macaulay, S. (2022). *For the children's sake: Foundations of education for home and school*. Crossway.
Shunya, A. (2017). *Ayurveda lifestyle wisdom: A complete prescription to optimize your health, prevent disease, and live with vitality and joy*. Sounds True.
Silberman, S. (2015). *NeuroTribes: The legacy of autism and the future of neurodiversity*. Avery.

Simone, R. (2010). *Aspergirls: Empowering females with Asperger syndrome*. Jessica Kingsley Publishers.

Stock Kranowitz, C. (2022). *The out-of-sync child: recognizing and coping with sensory processing disorder* (3rd ed.). TarcherPerigee.

Strasser, T. (1981). *The wave*. Ember.

The hero's journey in film. (n.d.). EduNut. Retrieved March 1, 2024, from https://vimeo.com/31320550

Thoreau, H. D., & Emerson, R. W. (2020). *Transcendentalists collection*.

Tieger, P. D., Barron-Tieger, B., & Tieger, K. (2018). *Do what you are: Discover the perfect career for you through the secrets of personality type*. Scribe Publications.

Tzu, L. (2010). *Tao te Ching*. Arcturus Publishing.

Villanueva, E. (2018). *Decolonizing wealth: Indigenous wisdom to heal divides and restore balance*. Berrett-Koehler Publishers.

Wrede, P. C. (2015). *Dealing with dragons*. Houghton Mifflin Harcourt.

Index

ADHD 30
Aspergers 12, 13, 155, 156, 158. See also autism, autistic.
Autism v, 12, 13, 77, 80, 84, 122, 128, 133, 136, 153, 156, 157
Autistic v, vii, 3, 4, 6, 7, 9, 12, 13, 47, 52, 77, 80, 82-84, 86, 96, 101, 102, 124, 127-129, 133, 134, 143, 156
Campbell, Joseph 37-45, 47, 117, 123, 155
Dehumanization 48, 49, 51
Down Syndrome 23, 80, 153
Dyscalculia 30, 113
Dysgraphia 30, 113, 156
Dyslexia 3, 30, 71-72, 113-114, 129, 135-136
Dyspraxia 113
Emerson, Ralph Waldo 17-18, 34, 158
Feuerstein, Reuven 67, 70
Hierarchy of Needs 28-37, 60, 105, 117, 120, 125, 154. See also Maslow, Abraham.
Horn, Dara 40-42, 48, 156
Humanities 41, 55-62
Hydroxyzine 89, 132, 154
Hyperlexia 6, 72, 114, 130, 135-136, 156
Indiana Jones 40, 84
Judaism 40-41, 57
Little Women 18, 34, 155
Logogens 71, 114
Maslow, Abraham 27-37, 41, 47, 60, 105, 108, 117, 120, 125, 153-154, 157. See also Hierarchy of Needs.
Mason, Charlotte 17-21, 23-28, 33, 37, 47, 55, 60, 65, 67, 70, 73, 75, 77, 83, 91, 96-98, 107-109, 115, 136, 143, 147-151, 156-157
Meltdown 3, 101-102
Montessori, Maria 17, 106, 157
Mythology 7, 37-42, 47, 53, 56, 155-156
Neuropsychology v, 5, 28, 106, 143
Nietzsche, Friedrich 17, 41-42, 157
Piaget, Jean p.65-68, 72, 137
Priestly Blessing 93-95, 98, 103
Rogers, Fred 9, 31, 93, 107, 157
Romanticism 18, 28

160 *Index*

Self-Actualization 29, 31-36, 117-125. *See also* Maslow, Abraham.
Sensory 3, 14, 24, 42, 69, 73, 76-77, 83-85, 88, 91, 102, 106-107, 128, 131, 137-138, 155, 158
Social 35, 66, 73, 84, 100, 107, 118-124, 131, 149
Special Needs vi-vii, 9, 13, 15, 138, 143, 145
Star Trek 14, 22, 40, 94
Thoreau, Henry David 17-18, 34, 158
Transcendence 33-36, 43, 47-48, 53, 61, 117-125. *See also* Maslow, Abraham.
Transcendentalism 17-18, 34, 158
Trauma 6, 49, 77, 83-85, 89, 95-96, 105-106, 124-125, 128, 131, 133, 157
Vygotsky, Lev 66-67, 69-71
Yoga 7, 34 38, 59, 88, 91, 97, 110, 120, 132, 155-156

This publication is designed to provide accurate and authoritative information in regard to the subject matter covered. It is sold with the understanding that neither the author nor the publisher is engaged in rendering legal, investment, accounting or other professional services. While the publisher and author have used their best efforts in preparing this book, they make no representations or warranties with respect to the accuracy or completeness of the contents of this book and specifically disclaim any implied warranties of merchantability or fitness for a particular purpose. No warranty may be created or extended by sales representatives or written sales materials. The advice and strategies contained herein may not be suitable for your situation. You should consult with a professional when appropriate. Neither the publisher nor the author shall be liable for any loss of profit or any other commercial damages, including but not limited to special, incidental, consequential, personal, or other damages.